R-4054-LACH

AIDS-Related Knowledge, Attitudes, Beliefs, and Behaviors in Los Angeles County

David E. Kanouse, Sandra H. Berry,
E. Michael Gorman, Elizabeth M. Yano,
Sally Carson, Allan Abrahamse

Prepared for the
AIDS Program Office,
Los Angeles County Department of Health Services

RAND

PREFACE

This report documents the results of a survey of the general public conducted for the AIDS Program Office, Los Angeles County Department of Health Services. The purposes of the survey were to provide information about the occurrence within the general population of Los Angeles County of sexual and drug-taking behaviors that can spread human immunodeficiency virus (HIV) infection and to determine the public's knowledge, attitudes, and opinions about the AIDS epidemic. This information may be used to guide programmatic efforts in planning effective education and prevention activities aimed at reducing the risk of HIV infection in the general public. The survey was conducted by telephone from October 1989 to January 1990 on a random sample of 1,305 residents of Los Angeles County. Black and Hispanic households were oversampled to obtain adequate information about ethnic populations in the county.

This survey was conducted concurrently with an AIDS-related survey of gay and bisexual men in Los Angeles County. Results from that survey are reported in:

> David E. Kanouse, Sandra H. Berry, E. Michael Gorman, Elizabeth M. Yano, and Sally Carson, *Response to the AIDS Epidemic: A Survey of Homosexual and Bisexual Men in Los Angeles County*, RAND, R-4031-LACH, 1991.

SUMMARY AND OVERVIEW

AIDS IN LOS ANGELES COUNTY

Los Angeles County has the second highest number of acquired immunodeficiency syndrome (AIDS) cases in the United States,[1] making AIDS and human immunodeficiency virus (HIV) disease major public health issues for the county. Although HIV infection has been primarily a disease of young adult males, the infection has now spread to women and children and across all age groups (CDC, 1990a; Los Angeles County DHS, 1990).[2]

AIDS also represents a particular risk among blacks and Hispanics, with AIDS cases among blacks outpacing their population representation in the county.[3] Nearly one in five (19 percent) of the AIDS cases diagnosed in Los Angeles County has been among Hispanics, with another 16 percent among black residents.

Even though the great majority of AIDS cases have occurred in homosexual and bisexual men, 12 percent of adults with AIDS in the county have some history of intravenous drug use. Among women with AIDS, heterosexual contact is an important mode of transmission: Nearly half of these women (47 percent) have no known history of IV drug use, with the remainder divided about equally between those who do (26 percent) and those whose drug use history is unknown (27 percent). Currently, the incidence of AIDS in California is increasing more rapidly among women than among men and more rapidly among heterosexual men than among gay/bisexual men (Capell et al., 1990).[4] These changing trends in AIDS incidence among those traditionally less at risk combined with the growing

[1]As of December 31, 1990, a cumulative total of 11,005 adult AIDS cases had been reported and confirmed by the Los Angeles County Department of Health Services.

[2]Although 62 percent of the cases have been diagnosed in men and women in their twenties and thirties, nearly one-quarter are in their forties and nearly another 10 percent are in their fifties.

[3]Hispanics account for a lower proportion of AIDS cases than they do of the county population, but their share of AIDS cases has been consistently growing.

[4]From November 1988 to November 1989, AIDS incidence increased 73 percent among women, 63 percent among heterosexual men, and 38 percent among gay/bisexual men (including intravenous drug users). Interpretation of these differential growth rates is not straightforward, since they may be affected by several factors, including differences between groups in reporting trends and access to treatment, and the "lag" that results from differences in the time when the virus became established in various subpopulations.

drug problems in Los Angeles County suggest that the AIDS virus may be gaining a foothold in more segments of the county's population.

Although AIDS has already exacted an enormous toll and may do so increasingly in the next several years, public health officials lack information that could be very useful in planning effective education and prevention efforts for the general population in Los Angeles County. Particularly little information is available about the prevalence of behaviors linked to HIV transmission in the general population or about the extent of the public's knowledge and perceptions of the risks associated with AIDS. Our aim is to describe and analyze the magnitude and patterns of risk behaviors that may place the general public at heightened risk of HIV transmission and to elucidate some of the possible barriers to reducing risk through either broad-based or targeted approaches. We hope that this report will prove useful in addressing the specific needs of segments of the population at greatest risk.

PURPOSES OF THE SURVEY

This survey was conducted to collect population-based information on the occurrence among Los Angeles County residents of sexual and drug-taking behaviors that can lead to HIV transmission, to identify the characteristics of those who are placing themselves and their partners at increased risk of acquiring HIV infection, and to measure public knowledge, attitudes, and beliefs about the AIDS epidemic.

To meet these objectives, we surveyed a broad-based sample of 1,305 Los Angeles County residents to determine their knowledge of HIV transmission, the degree to which they engaged in high-risk sexual and drug use behavior, and the perceptions, attitudes, and beliefs that may influence their behavior. This information serves not only to characterize the activities and perspectives of a cross-section of the general public but also to provide a baseline against which future responses to the epidemic may be measured.

Although national and state-level studies of the general population's responses to the AIDS epidemic have been conducted, few reflect local needs and concerns. These can vary both on account of epidemiological patterns (e.g., the relative importance of sexual transmission compared with IV drug use) and the types of constraints affecting the community's ability to respond (state laws, levels of public funding, availability of an infrastructure of community groups, etc.).

Few surveys attempt to characterize specific patterns of risk behavior that will shape the course of the epidemic in a particular site. Geographic variations in patterns of risk behavior have led to marked differences in the numbers and risk group profiles of AIDS cases in various locations. This report is designed to provide public health officials with information that will help them effectively counter the spread of HIV infection among the general public in Los Angeles County.

The survey addressed a wide range of issues related to HIV infection and AIDS. We asked questions about the following topics:

- **Risk Behavior**. The survey inquired in some detail about respondents' partner relationships and recent sexual practices, including use of condoms; the survey also inquired about their use of intravenous and nonintravenous drugs.
- **Knowledge About AIDS and HIV Transmission**. The survey assessed basic knowledge and beliefs about AIDS and HIV transmission. Respondents were asked about the major modes of transmission and the risks of acquiring HIV infection through casual contacts. Responses to these questions can reveal knowledge gaps that need to be addressed in education and prevention efforts.
- **Risk Perceptions**. Respondents were asked to rate the riskiness of various sexual practices that can lead to transmission of HIV. The survey also inquired about the risks that they believed AIDS poses to health care workers.
- **Self-Reported Behavior Change**. Respondents were asked about social or sexual behavior changes they may have made in response to the AIDS epidemic.
- **HIV Antibody Testing**. The survey asked whether respondents had been tested for antibodies to the AIDS virus, and if so, where, when, how often, and with what results.
- **Public Opinion**. Respondents were asked their opinions about key AIDS policy issues and programs, including AIDS education in schools, the safety of the blood supply, partner notification programs, and allocation of public funds for AIDS.

MAJOR FINDINGS AND CONCLUSIONS

The survey yielded a rich body of data on public knowledge, attitudes, beliefs, and behavior with respect to the AIDS epidemic in Los Angeles County. For the most part, the results are consistent with those of national surveys. The following findings stand out as especially important.

1. High-Risk Sexual Behavior. High-risk behavior can be thought of as having two components—the nature of the activity and the type of partner with whom it is performed. We found that nearly three-quarters of all sexually active respondents had recently engaged in one potentially high-risk behavior (vaginal intercourse without the protection of a condom); recent anal intercourse, with or without the protection of condoms, was reported by only 6 percent of these active respondents.

However, unprotected sex seldom occurred in the context of high-risk partner selection. In particular, very few county residents who participated in our survey reported current sexual involvement with multiple partners. Only 4 percent of those who were sexually active had sex with more than one person in the past four weeks, and 24 percent of sexually active respondents (those with at least one partner in the last five years) had no sex during that time. This is consistent with national surveys indicating that only 4–6 percent of married men aged 25–49 reported more than one sexual partner in the preceding 12 months (Turner et al., 1989a).

County residents do not normally use condoms, so the behaviors that many of them engage in could easily lead to infection with HIV and other pathogens if they have many partners (or ill-chosen ones). But even allowing for probable underrepresentation of high-risk people[5] and for underreporting of high-risk behavior, our survey results suggest a fairly low level of sexual "mixing," or partner turnover, in the population as a whole. If turnover is indeed low, then the HIV pathogen will not spread very rapidly within the overall population, even if most people do not use condoms. The incidence of new infections will tend instead to concentrate in demographic subgroups where sexual mixing is well above the population average (and where the virus is apt to be already well established).

2. Drug-Related Risk Behavior. This type of behavior is probably even more difficult than sexual behavior to capture accurately in a telephone interview; our data surely underrepresent those at greatest risk. Nearly a third of respondents had histories of recreational drug use, and 6 percent admitted to having used drugs within the last four weeks. But fewer than 2 percent acknowledged having taken drugs by injection, and only one respondent admitted doing so in the past

---

[5]A telephone survey misses altogether households without telephones and also fails to capture information from some people who are difficult to reach or uncooperative. These excluded or underrepresented groups are apt to include many high-risk people.

year. Clearly, use of injection drugs is extremely rare in the types of people we interviewed in our survey, and rare (though probably less so) in the population of all county residents. This finding is consistent with the epidemiological profile of reported AIDS cases in the county, in which IV drug use plays a much less prominent role than it does in several East Coast cities and in the United States as a whole.

Use of drugs or alcohol before or during sexual activity could increase the risk of HIV transmission by increasing the frequency of high-risk sex or decreasing participants' propensity to take precautions. For that reason, we asked how frequently alcohol or drugs were used in conjunction with sex. Very few people report using these substances in conjunction with sex regularly (7 percent for alcohol, about 4 percent for drugs). Because the county's population is so diverse, there may well be segments where such use is much more common, as it is in the gay/bisexual community (Kanouse et al., 1991).

3. Knowledge. The principal modes of transmission of HIV infection are now nearly universally known among county residents; knowledge of the low risk of casual transmission is not. Thus, the remaining knowledge gaps identified by our survey mainly concern casual transmission, suggesting a need for increasing the emphasis in public health messages on how AIDS is *not* spread as well as on how it is.

The high level of awareness of major transmission routes evidenced in our survey does not mean that public health education programs, having done their job, can go away. Continued dissemination of the message serves the critical function of maintaining public awareness of a lethal health risk that can be avoided through individual efforts. A sustained dissemination effort is also needed to educate young people as they become sexually active.

4. Perceived Risk. Seventy-eight percent of county residents who do not regularly use condoms do not believe that they and their partners are at risk of getting AIDS. As one might expect, this varied with marital and partnership status; but even among those not married or in a sexually exclusive relationship, two-thirds said that they and their partners were not at risk of AIDS and therefore do not use condoms.

Most people offered informed judgments of the risks associated with particular sexual behaviors. But knowledge of objective risks and judgments of personal risk can differ, and many Los Angeles County residents apparently see AIDS as a much greater risk for other people than it is for them or their sexual partners. For people whose behavior does place them at elevated risk, that perception can become a barrier to behavior change. Designing public health messages and interventions that counteract the tendency for those at risk to see that risk as threatening only other people is a challenge for the public health community.

5. Behavior Change. Among respondents who had been sexually active in the past ten years, 29 percent said that they made one or more changes in their behavior as a result of the AIDS epidemic. The most common changes had to do with partner choice—becoming more selective in the choice of sexual partners (24 percent) and reducing the total number of sexual partners or the number of casual partners (21 percent each). In addition, 16 percent of all respondents claimed to be using condoms more often, and 8 percent of the male respondents said that they had stopped having sex with prostitutes or hustlers. Although our survey did not attempt to measure respondents' recollections of their behavior before the AIDS epidemic, the percentages of people who report having made such changes are substantial in relation to the percentages who report currently engaging in them.

Many of those interviewed undoubtedly wish to appear to have responded in a socially desirable way to the epidemic, so the number of people who report having changed may exceed the number who have actually done so; but at a broader level, these results attest to a high level of public awareness of AIDS as a public health threat.

6. HIV Testing. We estimate that 23 percent of the county's adult population had been tested at least once for HIV infection by the time of the survey, compared to 21 percent of the nation's adult population (in a survey conducted at the same time). Since Los Angeles is one of the "epicenters" of the AIDS epidemic and facilities for anonymous testing have been available for some time, one might expect that the proportion tested in Los Angeles County would be above the national average.

The most common testing site was a Los Angeles County alternative test site (33 percent of those tested), followed by a private physician's office or a research center or hospital (about 25 percent for each). Men were more likely than women to seek testing, and those who knew someone with AIDS personally or professionally were especially likely to be tested. Although most people who have not yet been tested do not consider it likely that they will seek testing in the near future, 40 percent thought it at least somewhat likely that they would seek testing in the next six months, indicating a strong continuing demand for testing.

Fewer than one-half of 1 percent of respondents who had been tested were seropositive. On account of sample selection and participation biases that are inherent in all AIDS-related telephone surveys, our study does not offer a good basis for estimating a seropositivity rate for the countywide population.

7. Public Opinion. A majority of county residents express considerable concern about AIDS; most expect that it will be a bigger problem in the future. About half think they know someone who is at risk for AIDS, and almost a third know someone with AIDS. However, about 25 percent of respondents expressed reluctance to work with HIV-infected people, consistent with their beliefs that casual contact can transmit the virus.

Nearly all respondents expressed support for AIDS prevention education at the junior high and high school levels (98 percent) and at the elementary school level (87 percent). This represents nearly unanimous public approval of programs that have been the subject of considerable political controversy.

A majority believed that education programs aimed at specific risk groups (e.g., gay and bisexual men) are effective. There was also strong support for partner notification of those who test positive for HIV.

In allocating a hypothetical $100 of public funds, respondents gave priority to research on causes and cures of AIDS (45 percent) over prevention efforts (29 percent) and treatment (25 percent). This stands in contrast to actual spending, where treatment dominates.

ACKNOWLEDGMENTS

We are grateful to RAND colleagues Julie Brown, David Bryant, Laural Hill, Judy Perlman, and the Telephone Center staff for their assistance in designing and conducting a challenging survey on a sensitive topic. Larry Bye of Communications Technologies, Inc., consulted on instrument development. Frank Capell of the California Department of Health Services provided useful comments on a draft of the instrument. Daniel Relles and John Rolph provided helpful advice on statistical matters. Arleen Leibowitz and Jeffrey Wasserman supplied useful contextual material. Technical reviewers Howard Freeman and Anthony Pascal offered insightful critiques of a draft report. Joyce Peterson and Jerry Sollinger provided good advice on structuring and presentation. Janice Jones and Karin Suede provided capable text-processing assistance under tight deadline constraints. Richard Goldberg and Jonathan Freedman of the Los Angeles County Department of Health Services, AIDS Program Office, provided useful suggestions and support throughout the project. Finally, we are grateful to the many residents of Los Angeles County who provided us with detailed information about aspects of their lives that they do not often discuss, in the interest of contributing to a better understanding of the AIDS epidemic.

CONTENTS

FIGURES

TABLES

I. INTRODUCTION

We undertook this survey to measure AIDS-related knowledge, attitudes, beliefs, and behaviors of Los Angeles County adults. We conducted 1,305 interviews by telephone using random digit dial sampling procedures and a computer-assisted interview system. Interviews took about 25 minutes to complete and were conducted in English and Spanish. Interviewing was carried out from October to December 1989.

Although conducting a household telephone survey necessarily excludes some parts of the population from the sample, telephone coverage is generally high among Los Angeles residences; about 94 percent of households have telephones. The lower cost of telephone interviews compared with personal interviews allows for a much larger sample size for the same expenditure of resources. For these reasons we chose to conduct telephone interviews.

To select a probability sample of adults living in households (i.e., excluding persons in institutions such as dormitories, jails, hospitals, and others not part of households), we first selected a random sample of telephone numbers assigned to residences in Los Angeles County. We called these numbers and when we reached an eligible household we randomly selected one of the eligible adults in the household to respond to the interview. Below we briefly describe how we did this.

We began with lists of all area code and five-digit telephone prefixes assigned to Los Angeles County households.[1] From this list, two-digit numbers were randomly selected and attached to the area code and prefix combinations in proportion to the number of listed telephones known to be in service in each prefix. The randomly generated numbers included listed and unlisted numbers as well as numbers that were not working and numbers assigned to businesses and other nonhouseholds. The resulting list of numbers was randomly ordered and called by interviewers to determine the status of each number and to interview an individual in each eligible household.

A total of 4,049 numbers were sampled for this survey. This sample was selected in three parts. The first part was a sample of 2,982 numbers covering all of Los Angeles County, selected as described

[1]For Los Angeles, the area codes included 213, 818, 805, and 714. Prefixes with two or fewer working numbers out of the possible 100 numbers were excluded from selection.

above. The second part was a sample of 817 numbers chosen in the same way but limited to prefixes assigned to areas of the county where 85 percent of the households were black, according to the 1980 census. The third sample was similar to the second and consisted of 250 numbers selected from areas where between 82 and 95 percent of the households were Hispanic, according to the 1980 census. The black and Hispanic subsamples were selected to ensure that at least 300 black and 300 Hispanic interviews were completed. A simple random sample of the county would have yielded fewer black and Hispanic interviews than the county required for this survey. Of the 1,305 completed cases, 942 were from the random sample of the county, 283 were from the black subsample, and 80 were from the Hispanic subsample. Although not all cases in each of the subsamples were black or Hispanic, all of them were included in the sample we analyzed.

When an interviewer contacted someone by telephone, he or she first verified that the number was a household in Los Angeles County and then asked how many adults were living in the household who were between the ages of 18 and 75. If there was more than one, the interviewer asked to speak to the adult who had had the most recent birthday. Since birth dates are approximately randomly distributed, this provided a simple way of selecting randomly within the household.

The remainder of this report is organized as follows: Sec. II documents the sampling approach and methods used to conduct the survey; Sec. III presents study findings regarding knowledge, attitudes, beliefs, and behaviors. Section IV offers conclusions and discusses policy implications. An appendix provides detailed results of selected multivariate analyses.

II. THE SURVEY

SURVEY PROCEDURES AND OUTCOMES

Interviews were attempted seven days a week during the hours of 9 AM to 9 PM on weekdays, 10 AM to 6 PM on Saturdays, and noon to 8 PM on Sundays. Assignment of telephone numbers to interviewers was controlled by computer, so that each number was attempted during the day, in the evening, and on weekends. Over 20,000 calls were made to complete the survey, up to a maximum of 15 calls per case.[1]

The interview was available in English and Spanish; both versions were programmed into the computer-assisted telephone interviewing system, and interviewers could use the version respondents found most comfortable to answer. Whenever possible, we assigned bilingual interviewers to attempt cases in areas where Spanish-speaking respondents were most likely to be found. However, when an English-speaking interviewer encountered a Spanish-speaking person and could not communicate with him or her, the case was assigned for callbacks by Spanish-speaking interviewers. Altogether, 155 interviews were carried out in Spanish.

Table 1 shows the disposition of sampled cases. Of the 4,050 numbers sampled, 1,662 were ineligible either because they were not working numbers, they belonged to businesses, or there was no eligible respondent in the household (e.g., those contacted were too young or too old). Of the remaining 2,388 eligible cases, we completed interviews with 1,305, for a completion rate of 55 percent. The 1,083 eligible cases that were not completed included 68 partial completes, 154 refusals to be interviewed, 122 refusals to screen for eligibility, 82 language problems (not English or Spanish), and 13 cases where the selected respondent was away or too ill to be interviewed (see Table 1). In the remaining 644 eligible cases, we were simply unable to complete an interview (but had not received a refusal) by the time the field period ended; the principal reasons were that respondents were not at home, had answering machines, or did not keep appointments for the interview. Completion rates were slightly lower (49 percent) in the Hispanic subsample and higher (62 percent) in the black subsample than in the random sample (55 percent).

---

[1]Multiple callbacks may be especially important to reduce bias in surveys on the prevalence of risky sexual behavior, since the evidence suggests that those who are difficult to reach by telephone are more likely to engage in such behavior (Capell and Schiller, 1989).

Table 1

DISPOSITION OF CASES IN RANDOM DIGIT DIAL SAMPLE

Disposition	Number of Cases	Percent of Cases
Ineligible Numbers		
Confirmed not working	902	22.3
No answer 15+ rings	79	2.0
Business	513	12.7
Not private residence	7	0.0
No eligible respondent	136	3.3
Other ineligible[a]	25	0.6
Total	1,662	41.0
Presumed Eligible Household Numbers—Not Screened		
Household refused to screen	122	3.0
Language problem	50	1.2
In progress at end of study	262	6.5
Other eligible not screened[b]	38	0.9
Total	472	11.6
Screened Eligible Household Numbers		
Selected respondent refused interview	154	3.8
Language problem	32	0.8
Unavailable or ill	13	0.3
In progress at end of study	344	8.5
Completed interview	1,305	32.2
Partial complete	68	1.7
Total	1,916	47.3
Total no. attempted	4,050	100.0

[a]Includes cases outside Los Angeles County, car phones, pay phones, computer lines and telephones in institutions, vacant residences, etc.

[b]Includes non-business answering machines, lines for the disabled, and temporarily out-of-service residential numbers.

Although statewide surveys on AIDS-related issues have achieved higher response rates (Capell and Schiller, 1989), this response rate compares favorably with rates for similar surveys in the Los Angeles area. For example, a survey about AIDS-related risk behaviors conducted with Los Angeles County men in 1988 achieved a 45 percent response rate (Freeman et al., 1989). And a countywide telephone survey conducted by RAND in 1988 that elicited public opinion about quality of life in Los Angeles obtained a 54 percent response rate (Berry, 1988).

In general, telephone survey completion rates in Los Angeles tend to be somewhat lower than the national average. According to a national sampling firm, Los Angeles is the third least cooperative area of the country for interviewing (after Miami and Ft. Lauderdale); 61 percent of its residential numbers are unlisted—the second highest rate in the nation and twice the national average. We asked respondents whether we had reached them on a listed or unlisted number. Because only 36 percent reported being reached on an unlisted number, we assume that our response rate was lower among people with unlisted telephones.

SAMPLING ADJUSTMENTS

In analyzing sample surveys, the goal is for each sample element to have a probability of having entered the sample that represents its actual frequency in the population, so it is sometimes necessary to correct for factors in the sampling and field process that alter that probability. In this survey, we corrected for the unequal sampling probabilities associated with households of unequal size and with having more than one telephone line. We also adjusted for selection factors associated with major demographic characteristics, such as gender, race, and ethnicity.[2] This included a correction for the effects of intentionally oversampling blacks and Hispanics. These corrections are described briefly below.

Since households are sampled through telephone lines, a household with two telephone lines (two separate telephone numbers) is twice as likely to enter the sample as a household with one line. If it has three lines, it has three times the chances of entering the sample, etc. At the end of the interview we asked each respondent for the number of telephone lines going into his household and used that information to adjust our sample weights. Two-hundred and forty-nine households had more than one telephone line.

Within each sampled household, there may be one or more eligible person. If only one person is eligible, that person has a 100 percent chance of being selected for the interview. If two people are eligible, each has a 50 percent chance of being selected, etc. Since the unit of analysis in this survey is the individual, it is necessary to correct for the fact that individual respondents have had different chances of

[2]Although we did not intentionally oversample women, they were more likely than men to complete interviews; we used an adjustment to correct for this.

being selected, and we have done so in this analysis by adjusting for household size.

In addition to the corrections necessitated by the requirements of telephone sampling methodology, we also adjusted for two factors caused by differences in household composition and differences in willingness to participate. These are (1) we reached more females than males in the telephone survey sample and (2) the race and ethnicity distribution among those we reached differs from the projected race and ethnicity distribution of Los Angeles County. In particular, we reached a larger proportion of whites who were not Hispanic than of Hispanics, blacks, and Asians. This is common in telephone interviewing and can happen for a number of reasons, including differences in the distribution of single compared with multiple adult households across males, females, and racial/ethnic groups, differences in our ability to reach these households by telephone, and differences in their willingness to participate in a telephone interview. Therefore, we adjusted (or "weighted") the sample to reflect the age-specific gender, race, and ethnicity distribution projected by the Los Angeles County Department of Regional Planning for 1990. Our adjusted distribution is 43 percent white, 10 percent black, 33 percent Hispanic, and 13 percent Asian and other.

Finally, as noted, we selected not only a random sample of the entire county but also two subsamples—one of predominantly black and one of predominantly Hispanic respondents. This was done to ensure adequate sample sizes of these minorities, but it raised the question of whether and how to combine this information in analyses of the countywide population. One option was to analyze each sample separately, but that would have reduced the possibilities for making useful comparisons among the racial/ethnic groups; effective comparisons can be made only within the random component of the sample, and the numbers of blacks and Hispanics are small. An alternative was to combine the three samples for the analysis, adjusting for the differences between the demographic composition of this combined sample and the countywide demographic composition by assigning lower weights to cases from the two subsamples. This was attractive in that it would make use of all the data, but the projected countywide results could be distorted from those of a simple random countywide sample if the black and Hispanic cases from the oversampled areas were much different from the black and Hispanic cases obtained in a random countywide sample.

We chose to employ both options and compare the results. In both cases, we weighted the observations in the sample to reflect the race/ethnicity distribution of the county projected for the year 1990.

The differences in results between the two samples were very small (on the order of 1 percent) for all analyses, so we have chosen to present the results from the combined sample to take advantage of the larger number of cases.

As described, we have adjusted the sample weights to correct for known sources of potential bias in our sample to increase the accuracy of the results of this survey. But these weighting adjustments are not a perfect substitute for actually obtaining a random sample of that population. Since slightly fewer than half the eligible households we identified did not cooperate, it is very likely that the households that did cooperate differ from those that did not.[3] Without information about the nonrespondents, however, we cannot assess the magnitude or the direction of these differences in our sample.[4] Clearly, these problems and limitations need to be kept in mind in interpreting study results.

DESCRIPTION OF THE SURVEY POPULATION

Table 2 describes the weighted sample population. Fifty-one percent of the weighted sample are female and 49 percent male. Just under half the sample (47 percent) were age 35 or younger and just over a quarter (27 percent) were age 50 and over. The racial/ethnic breakdown is 43 percent white, 10 percent black, 33 percent Hispanic, 9 percent Asian, and about 5 percent mixed and other races.

Nearly 70 percent of the respondents were working full- or part-time or had a job but were not working on account of vacation or illness. About 5 percent were unemployed or laid off, and 11 percent were retired. The rest were in school, keeping house, or otherwise outside the labor force. About 18 percent of the sample had not finished high school, 29 percent were high school graduates, 25 percent had some college, and 27 percent were college graduates. About 34 percent of the respondents reported household incomes of less than $20,000, about 33 percent had incomes of $20,000–$49,999, and 33 percent had household incomes of $50,000 or more.

It is difficult to assess how the demographic characteristics of our sample compare to those of the 1990 county adult population, since

[3]Research Triangle Institute (1990) found that nonrespondents from the first round of interviewing who were later persuaded to cooperate had significantly higher self-reported rates of risk behavior.

[4]Surveys addressing human sexual behavior face formidable difficulties in collecting highly sensitive information. For discussions of some of these difficulties, see Catania et al. (1990a, 1990b), Green and Wiener (1980), and Miller et al. (1990).

Table 2

PERCENTAGE DISTRIBUTION OF RESPONDENTS' DEMOGRAPHIC CHARACTERISTICS, WEIGHTED TO THE POPULATION

Characteristic	Distribution	Characteristic	Distribution
Education		Employment	
No high school diploma	18	Employed full- or part-time	70
High school diploma	29	Unemployed, laid off	5
Some college	25	Retired, disabled	11
College graduate	15	Other not working	14
Some graduate training	12		
Age		Household Income	
18–24	20	Less than $10,000	4
25–34	23	$10,000–$19,999	30
35–44	20	$20,000–$34,999	19
45–54	15	$35,000–$49,999	14
55–64	13	$50,000–$99,999	29
65 and older	9	$100,000 or more	4
Race/ethnicity		Gender	
White	43	Male	49
Black	10	Female	51
Hispanic	33		
Asian	9		
Mixed/other	5		

the latter can only be estimated. The most comprehensive data source, the 1980 census, is outdated, and the results of the 1990 census are now being tabulated and county information will not be available for some time. Other available sources do not provide the same demographic breakdowns used in our study or are for a somewhat different population.

We believe that our survey is representative of the range of the variation in the county population, subject to the biases found in other telephone surveys—namely, lower response rates among older and less well-educated respondents. In addition, the random selection of a respondent within households means that the most knowledgeable respondent may not be reporting some of the information. In particular, household income may not be as accurately reported by a teenager in the household as it would have been by the parent.

III. RESULTS

SEXUAL RISK BEHAVIOR IN THE GENERAL PUBLIC

Background

Although AIDS in Los Angeles County still occurs predominantly among homosexual and bisexual men, incidence trends show substantial increases among heterosexual men and women. Rates of infection among intravenous drug users (IVDUs) and the heterosexual partners of those already infected[1] have steadily grown, and such cases now constitute an increasing share of new AIDS cases. Although the diffusion of the AIDS epidemic into the heterosexual community has been slow rather than explosive as had been feared, the increase should not be viewed lightly.

The risk of acquiring HIV infection depends on three things: (1) the degree to which people engage in behaviors linked to HIV transmission, (2) the prevalence of HIV infection in the population, and (3) the pattern of contacts (via high-risk behaviors) between those infected and those not yet infected.[2] This survey was designed to address only the first of these three factors. The second factor, the prevalence of HIV infection in Los Angeles County, is not known but can be estimated in various ways, as described below. The third, extent of contact between those infected and those who are susceptible through high-risk behavior, is largely unknown.

Only limited information is available on the sexual practices of the general population, especially outside of established relationships. More data are needed on sexual relations that occur outside of marriage and on variations in sexual practices across different types of partners (Turner et al., 1989b). This is a highly sensitive topic, which may explain why it has often been avoided altogether in many of the

---

[1]Sexual partners of individuals who have already been infected with the AIDS virus especially include women who have had sexual contact with IVDUs or with bisexual men.

[2]This differs from the first factor in that it refers to patterns of partner selection rather than sexual activity per se. If infection is initially concentrated in a subpopulation whose sexual contacts occur mostly within the group rather than with other groups, the epidemic will spread much more slowly outside that subpopulation than it would if groups mixed more freely. In this case of segregated patterns of sexual contact, people's chances of getting infected depend not only on their sexual behavior but on which sexual "group" they are in.

AIDS-related surveys conducted in the United States.[3] This dearth of information forms a serious barrier to our understanding of the patterns of behavior that place the public at risk of HIV infection or other sexually transmitted diseases.[4]

Prevalence of HIV Infection in Los Angeles County

Most of the available data on HIV prevalence come from a surveillance system developed by the Centers for Disease Control (CDC) that includes ongoing surveys of segments of the population and sentinel hospital surveillance efforts in selected areas of the country (for a description of the family of surveys that this system comprises, see Pappaioanou et al., 1990). Routine HIV testing of blood donors, newborn infants in participating hospitals, and military applicants also provides useful data, especially for tracking trends in infection rates over time. However, the samples are not representative and cannot be generalized to the local or national populations.[5]

In Los Angeles County in 1989, 49,354 newborns were tested for HIV antibodies (a positive test indicates that the *mother* is infected with HIV); 39 tested seropositive, for a rate of 0.078 percent, close to the statewide rate of 0.074 percent.[6]

Of military applicants tested in Los Angeles from October 1985 through September 1990, 0.22 percent tested seropositive, compared with 0.16 percent in California and 0.09 percent nationwide.

Confidential HIV testing is available at Los Angeles County–University of Southern California Women's Hospital, at 20 drug treatment centers, and in juvenile detention facilities. A total of 22,880 persons accepted HIV testing in this program during 1990, of whom 499 (2.2 percent) tested HIV seropositive. Blinded serosurveys are

[3]Several AIDS-related surveys conducted by national, state, and local agencies and organizations have limited themselves to AIDS-related knowledge and attitudes (e.g., Hardy, 1990a, 1990b). This is perhaps understandable considering the furor raised by the prospect of a national household survey of sexual behavior, whose funding was quashed before the survey could be implemented.

[4]For several years, rates of syphilis and gonorrhea infection have been higher in Los Angeles County than in most other large metropolitan areas, so that public health officials and the public have other good reasons besides HIV infection to be concerned about sexually transmitted diseases.

[5]A national household-based survey of HIV seroprevalence was long under consideration, but plans for such a survey have been scrapped following analysis of results from a feasibility study, which indicated that substantial resources and extensive community preparation would be needed to implement such a survey (CDC, 1991; RTI, 1990).

[6]Seroprevalence figures for the county were provided by the AIDS Program Office, Los Angeles County Department of Health Services.

conducted in methadone maintenance/detoxification clinics, sexually transmitted disease (STD) clinics, tuberculosis clinics, and family planning and prenatal care clinics. Seroprevalence rates at methadone treatment clinics were 1.6 percent in 1988, 2.3 percent in 1989, and 2.0 percent in 1990. Among drug users not in treatment (tested at alternative test sites, STD clinics, jails, homeless shelters, and public places), seropositivity rates range from 5 to 10 percent.

During the first half of 1990, 8,324 persons were tested anonymously in state-funded alternative test sites; 5.7 percent were seropositive. During the last half of 1990, seropositivity rates for 2,725 persons tested in STD clinics were 3.9 percent, 2.2 percent, and 3.8 percent among whites, blacks, and Latinos, respectively.[7] In tuberculosis clinics, 8.0 percent of 138 patients tested seropositive. Of 2,026 women of reproductive age who underwent confidential testing in a family planning or a prenatal clinic, only one tested seropositive.

As these figures show, the prevalence of HIV infection varies markedly among various subpopulations in Los Angeles County. This marked variation is possible both because of the extreme inefficiency of transmission of HIV through casual contact and because the risk behaviors that spread HIV infection occur with much greater frequency in some groups.

Previous Population-Based Studies of Sexual Behavior

Much of our current knowledge of sexual behavior derives from Kinsey data of nearly 50 years ago, but a handful of studies since then offer insights into behavioral patterns in the general public. Few are population-based; most rely instead on convenience samples in public health clinics or colleges,[8] magazine readership surveys, or supplements to surveys on other topics.[9] However informative they may be about the particular sample studied, these surveys permit few conclusions about the overall population.

---

[7]Seropositivity rates varied by risk group as well; 38 percent of 103 homosexual males, 15 percent of 141 bisexual males, 67 percent of six homosexual male intravenous drug users, and 4 percent of 125 heterosexual male intravenous drug users tested seropositive.

[8]For example, DeBuono and colleagues (1990) studied women at a university student health service in the Northwest, and Landefeld et al. (1988) studied college students in an outpatient facility in Ohio to determine the degree to which the students were sexually active and how many sexual partners they had had.

[9]For example, Biggar and colleagues (reported in Turner et al., 1989b) asked successive cohorts of women who had served as healthy controls in a cancer study in five metropolitan areas in the United States about the number of sexual partners they had had in the past decade. Although these controls may have been adequate for the purposes of the comparisons made in the cancer study, there is no way to tell how they relate to women in general or even to women in these metropolitan areas.

To glean information from the most representative samples available, members of the National Research Council (Turner et al., 1989b) combined and analyzed data from two surveys that asked about the number of sexual partners people had had in the past year. These surveys were (1) the General Social Survey (or GSS) conducted in 1988 through a collaboration between the National Institute of Child Health and Development (NICHD) and the National Opinion Research Center (NORC)[10] and (2) a *Los Angeles Times* telephone survey conducted in 1987.[11]

Several important findings emerge from the combined results of these surveys:

1. Among unmarried men and women ages 18–24, 19 percent of the women and 16 percent of the men reported having had no sexual partners in the entire year and 15 percent of women and 40 percent of men had had three or more partners in the past year (this percentage declined with age among men).
2. Among unmarried men and women of all ages, 6 percent of men and 1 percent of women reported having had nine or more sexual partners in the past year.
3. Among married men and women ages 25–49, from 4–6 percent of men and from 1–2 percent of the women had had two or more sexual partners in the past year.

These data suggest that a fairly large proportion of the population, including most married men and women and perhaps a fifth or a sixth of all unmarried men and women, are at little or no risk of acquiring HIV infection through their sexual behavior during the course of a given year. These people are either abstinent or are mutually monogamous with a single sexual partner (who is likely in most cases to be uninfected). At the same time, the data suggest that there are pockets of sexually active men and women who face added risk of HIV infection through the sheer number of sexual partners they have.

---

[10]The GSS is a full probability sample survey of noninstitutionalized adults in the United States that is conducted annually through the auspices of NICHD/NORC. In 1988, 1,481 adults were interviewed (77 percent response rate) regarding social and political topics, after which they completed a one-page self-administered survey asking about the number, gender, and relationships with sexual partners over the previous 12 months.

[11]The *Los Angeles Times* surveyed 2,095 adults from a national probability sample of telephone-owning households, oversampling households in five major metropolitan areas. Low response rates severely limited the ability to project estimates of behavior to the entire adult population, as intended, but the survey does provide important information on adults who may be reached by telephone and who consent to a public opinion survey. Although response rates were low, refusals were based on willingness to participate in any survey (over 90 percent refused during household screening), not on the fact that the survey covered AIDS or sexual behavior in particular.

The council also reviewed another study of sexual behavior of black and white women in Los Angeles (Wyatt, 1985). Compared to the GSS and *Los Angeles Times* surveys, this survey captured a smaller and probably a more specialized sample of women.[12] Wyatt found that 39 percent of white women and 48 percent of black women had had their first sexual intercourse by the age of 16 and that 74 percent of white women and 26 percent of black women had had 13 or more sexual partners since the age of 18. Further, 43 percent of white women and 21 percent of black women reported "some" experience with anal intercourse, while 5 to 6 percent engaged in it at least once a month. Although selection factors must surely have played a part in respondents' willingness to cooperate in such a long interview,[13] these results underscore that there are indeed people in the county who are sexually very active and who engage in behaviors that place them at increased risk of HIV infection.

How We Measured Sexual Behavior

Our goals required explicit and detailed information on sexual behavior. At the same time, our survey respondents were quite diverse both in their behavior and in their sensitivity to many of the questions posed. To fit the line of questioning to reported behavior, we tailored questions to specific subgroups of respondents defined by marital/partnership status and sexual behavior in recent years.

First, we determined the respondent's marital status (married, divorced, separated, widowed, or never married).[14] If the respondent indicated that he or she was not currently married, we asked about

---

[12]Two probability samples were drawn of 18- to 36-year-old white (n = 122) and black women (n = 126), matched on education, marital status, and the presence of children in the household. Respondents were recruited by telephone survey for an in-person structured interview that took from three to eight hours to complete. The refusal rate was 45 percent.

[13]Willingness to participate in a survey of sexual behavior is greater among individuals who are relatively comfortable talking about intimate behavior. To the extent that such comfort is related to sexual experience, this will lead to an overrepresentation of people with more experience. Moreover, among those who may be especially willing to participate in an hours-long interview are those with a strong personal interest in the topic of the research (in this case, sexual abuse). Because of the small sample sizes, the likelihood of unusual selection biases, and the unusual pattern of the results compared to other general population surveys we have reviewed, we believe that these results reflect a specialized segment rather than a broad cross-section of the population.

[14]A "single" category (for respondents who would not be more specific) was combined with the "never married" category. Although this may lead to a certain amount of misclassification (e.g., some recently divorced people may choose to label themselves single rather than divorced, for reasons outside our control or ability to study), our interest was in the respondent's classification of relationship status. As it happened, only 1.7 percent of the respondents selected the "single" category.

current involvement in some other type of primary relationship, defined as having "someone with whom you are intimately involved and feel particularly close to." Whether or not the respondent was married, we inquired about the gender of the partner,[15] the duration of the relationship, and the degree to which the relationship was exclusive or monogamous. We ascertained the exclusivity of the respondent's relationship by reading a series of categories and asking the respondent to select the category that "to the best of your knowledge . . . best describes your primary relationship." The categories were (1) neither of us has sex with other people, (2) only (he/she) has sex with other people, (3) only I have sex with other people, or (4) we both have sex with other people.

We refrained from asking detailed sexual behavior questions of respondents who said that they had never engaged in sexual relations or that they no longer did so. We therefore included two items designed to identify respondents who had not had any sexual partners in the past five or ten years, as explained in more detail below.[16] These items were directed at respondents who indicated they were neither married nor in another type of primary relationship.[17] Responses to these items determined the eligibility of these respondents for other behavioral items. Those who had not had sex in the past ten years skipped past all behavioral items (including HIV-testing behavior) since, for the most part, their sexual activity would have predated the HIV epidemic. Those who had not had any sexual partners in the past five years but had had sex in the past ten were questioned about their perceptions of the risk associated with different sexual behaviors and about the extent to which they had changed their behavior in response to the AIDS epidemic. This skip-pattern logic enabled us to capture information about respondents who had, in fact, changed the extent to which they engaged in sexual relations once the syndrome was recognized.

Of all remaining respondents (i.e., those who had had a sexual partner in the past five years), we asked a series of questions about

---

[15]Gender of partner in married relationships proved useful, in that a small number of the married respondents indicated marriage with a same sex partner.

[16]For the self-identified gay/bisexual men who were a part of our general population sample, we used a different criterion to determine eligibility for the behavioral items, identifying as eligible those who had had at least one sexual partner in the past 12 months.

[17]Since the survey was designed to examine the potential for HIV transmission, we elected to focus on the extent of historical sexual activity (e.g., "have you had any sexual partners in the past ten years?") among people who reported no current sexual partner. We did not seek similar historical information from married or other respondents reporting current sexual involvement.

their recent sexual experiences. Four-week recall periods were used for all sexual behavior items. These included:

- The number of different sexual partners during that time.
- Whether the respondent had had sex with a prostitute or hustler and, if so, how many times.[18]
- The frequency with which they had engaged in various sexual practices with their primary partner (or all of their partners if they reported more than one sexual partner in the past four weeks).[19]
- Vaginal intercourse with a condom.
- Vaginal intercourse without a condom.
- Anal intercourse with a condom.
- Anal intercourse without a condom.
- Oral sex with a condom.
- Oral sex without a condom.

Four-week recall periods were used to assure a reasonable likelihood that respondents could accurately recall their behavior. Some other studies have used "window" periods of longer duration (e.g., two months, six months, one year, a lifetime). Others have used a similarly short recall period to derive behavioral estimates for more prolonged periods; for example, they assume that behaviors reported during the four-week period occur at a steady rate and multiply by the desired number of months.

For the most part, prevalence estimates provided in this report rely on the four-week recall period as a cross-sectional view of behavior in Los Angeles County. Behavior is averaged across respondents to give as representative a view as possible of the total frequency of various types of sexual activity during a well-defined time period. For the individual respondent, however, the four-week period of reported activity may sometimes be atypical. This does not bias the cross-

[18]If a respondent reported sex with a prostitute or hustler in the past four weeks, we asked whether such partners were included in the number of sexual partners that the respondent had reported during that time. If not, the count was corrected and the interviewer proceeded to the next question.

[19]Some of the men in our general population sample identified themselves as homosexual or bisexual following a screening item that was asked of all men who indicated that they were married or in another primary relationship with a man. These respondents were asked a series of sexual behavior questions that differed from those asked other respondents in this general population survey, but that was identical to those asked of participants in a parallel study of behavior among homosexual and bisexual men in Los Angeles County (Kanouse et al., 1991). Since these men are also part of our general population survey, differences in the questions they were asked are considered in our presentation of the findings.

sectional view of behavior in the aggregate, because the atypically active periods captured for some respondents will tend to be balanced by the atypically inactive periods captured for other respondents.

Instability of individual patterns does pose problems, however, when we try to estimate the proportion of individuals who behave in a particular way over longer periods of time, because some of these individuals may (for want of opportunity, perhaps) not behave that way during a given four-week period (see Table 3).

We report the prevalence of each sexual behavior as the mean number of acts over the previous four weeks for all respondents reporting at least one sexual partner in the past five years. Since this includes respondents who have not been sexually active in the previous four weeks, it understates the extent to which those who are *currently active* engage in each behavior. Accordingly, we report the percentage of people engaging in each behavior to place the reported mean in context.

Partner Relationships

Over half of the sample reported being currently married (53 percent), and 30 percent reported having never been married. The remainder were divorced (9 percent), widowed (4 percent), or separated (4 percent). Among respondents who reported not being currently married (47 percent of the sample), nearly half (45 percent) reported being involved in another type of primary relationship.

Table 3

PERCENTAGE DISTRIBUTION OF RESPONDENTS' SEXUAL PARTNERS DURING THE PAST FOUR WEEKS AMONG THOSE SEXUALLY ACTIVE IN THE PAST FIVE YEARS

No. of Partners	Distribution
None	24.3
One	71.9
Two	2.3
Three	1.0
Four	0.1
Five	0.1
Six	0.3

NOTE: Percentages are weighted totals based on the responses of 1,136 men and women who reported having had sex in the previous five years.

Thus, three-quarters of the sample were currently involved in some type of relationship (Fig. 1). Among the 25 percent who did not have a primary partner, many were sexually active nonetheless. The extent to which men and women reported being involved in relationships differed slightly, with women reporting being either married or not involved more often than men.[20]

Ninety percent of respondents reported being monogamous in the relationships they had established. Of the 10 percent reporting nonexclusive relationships, only 2 percent reported that both partners

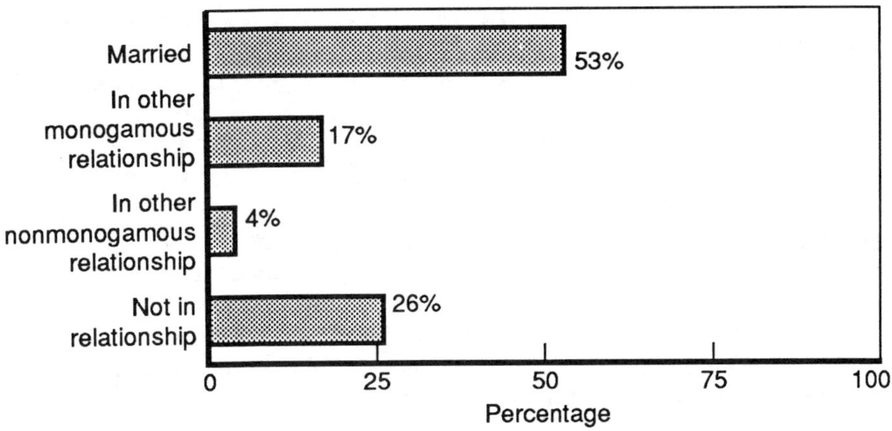

NOTE: Marital status was asked of all respondents (n = 1,305). Those not currently married (n = 710) were asked about their involvement in some other type of primary relationship (n = 386 not in a relationship). Those in a primary relationship (n = 321) were in turn asked about the exclusivity of the relationship with their primary partner. Percentages are weighted to the county population.

Fig. 1—Primary relationships of respondents

---

[20]Chi-square (4 d.f.) = 11.0, $p < 0.05$. To distinguish between opposite-sex and same-sex relationships, we also categorized relationships according to whether respondents were married, in a primary relationship, or uninvolved, and by the partners' gender. Patterns for men and women did not differ significantly: married to a member of opposite sex (51 percent for men compared with 53 percent for women), married to a member of same sex (0.1 percent for men compared with 1.1 percent for women), in a primary relationship with a member of opposite sex (22 percent for men compared with 19 percent for women), in a primary relationship with member of same sex (2 percent for men compared with 0.5 percent for women), and not in any type of primary relationship (25 percent for men compared with 27 percent for women).

were sexually active with other people.[21] Of course, some respondents may have been unaware of their partner's sexual activity outside the relationship. If we assume that respondent's partners could just as easily have been selected into the study as the respondents themselves, and that partners, if interviewed, would report sex outside the relationship at the same rate as did our respondents, then the results suggest that perhaps an additional 2 percent of respondents have partners who would report outside sexual activity of which our respondent is unaware.[22] Thus, the results imply an actual rate of nonexclusive behavior of about 12 percent, assuming no over- or underreporting of one's own outside sexual activity and no overreporting of one's partner's.[23] Unmarried men and women did not differ in the extent to which they reported being exclusive within primary relationships.[24]

Because of the higher risk of HIV transmission associated with male homosexual behavior, we asked all male respondents whether they had had sex with other men.[25] Only 2 percent of the male respondents indicated having done so within the past ten years. We also examined the degree to which respondents reported same-sex pairings in their relationships. Fewer than 1 percent of the men considered themselves married to other men, and about 1 percent of the women reported themselves currently married to other women. About 1.5 percent of the men reported being in a primary relationship with a man and 0.5 percent of the women reported being in a primary relationship with a woman.

Number of Sexual Partners

We asked all respondents who had had at least one sexual partner in the past five years about the number of sexual partners they had

[21]Respondents reported both partners having sex outside the relationship (2 percent), only the respondent having sex outside the relationship (5 percent), and only the other partner having sex outside the relationship (3 percent).

[22]This is the difference between the 5 percent who report that only they have outside sex and the 3 percent who report that only their partners have outside sex.

[23]This is in sharp contrast to findings in the companion report (Kanouse et al., 1991) among gay/bisexual men where 40 percent of the respondents reported that one or both partners have sex outside the relationship.

[24]Three percent of women and 5 percent of men reported that one or both partners were not exclusive (chi-square (3 d.f.) = 5.9, p = 0.12).

[25]Men were asked to state which category best described them: category A, men who have had sex with other men, even if it was only once or twice, within the past ten years or category B, men who have had sex only with women, or have not had sex at all, within the past ten years.

had in the past four weeks.[26] Nearly one-quarter (24 percent) reported having had no sexual partners in the previous four-week period. The vast majority reported having only one partner; only 4 percent reported two or more partners during the four-week period before the interview. No one reported having more than six partners in the previous four-week period (see Table 3).

These results are consistent with those of recent national surveys, which indicate that only a small proportion of *married* men and women have more than one partner during a 12-month period (Miller et al., 1990, pp. 474–475). However, these surveys also show much higher proportions of *unmarried* men and women in younger age groups having multiple partners during a 12-month period. For example, about 35 percent of unmarried men and 22 percent of unmarried women between the ages of 25 and 34 reported having had more than one partner during the preceding 12 months. The time frame used in our study is much shorter, so our results cannot directly be compared with results of these national surveys. It is possible that many people who have multiple partners over a year's time never have more than one during a given month. A pattern of "serial monogamy" with a high rate of turnover in partners would lead to quite different patterns of results for the short term compared with the long term.

Of those reporting one or more partners in the past four weeks, fewer than 1 percent reported having had a partner who was a prostitute or hustler.[27] Since population-based data on the use of female prostitutes are virtually nonexistent, it is difficult to place this number in perspective. As we shall see, however, a much larger proportion of men reported that they had stopped going to prostitutes as a result of the AIDS epidemic.

---

[26]As described above, all respondents who indicated that they were neither married nor presently involved in some other type of primary relationship were asked whether they had had a sexual partner in the past ten years. Twenty-nine percent of the people who were not in any type of relationship said that they had not had a sexual partner for at least ten years. Of the remaining 71 percent who had such a partner, 9 percent had not had a sexual partner in the past five years. None of these respondents were asked any of the sexual behavior items, including the number of sexual partners. Roughly 12 percent of the total sample had been sexually inactive for five years or more.

[27]We asked all respondents about contacts with prostitutes or hustlers; those reporting such contacts were all men.

Patterns of Sexual Activity in Los Angeles County

Respondents who reported at least one sexual partner in the past four weeks were asked about specific sexual practices. We present the results two ways. First, we report the percentage of people who said that they had engaged in a particular sexual behavior at all during the four-week period. Second, we report the mean frequency with which they engaged in that behavior during the four-week period.

We focus on what we refer to as "unprotected" intercourse, by which we mean oral, genital, or anal intercourse without the use of condoms. Condoms are the preferred barrier method for preventing transmission of all sexually transmitted disease agents, including HIV. Because we are interested in prophylaxis rather than contraception, we did not inquire about respondents' use of other forms of contraceptives, such as diaphragms, birth control pills, and IUDs. It should be recognized, however, that decisions regarding condom use may be affected by contraceptive as well as prophylactic concerns.

Among the (recently) sexually active respondents who were asked about specific practices, nearly three-quarters (72 percent) had engaged in unprotected vaginal intercourse (by the foregoing definition) at least once in a given four-week period, three times the proportion who used condoms (24 percent). Almost one-third (31 percent) reported engaging in oral-genital sex at least once in the past four weeks, with only 4 percent reporting oral sex using condoms.

Only 4 percent of these active respondents said that they had recently engaged in unprotected anal intercourse—probably the riskiest practice with respect to the likelihood of HIV transmission if the insertive partner is infected. An even smaller number (2 percent) reported anal intercourse using condoms (Fig. 2).

Despite public knowledge and concern about HIV infection, condom use is infrequent. Condoms are used by roughly a third of those engaging in anal intercourse, a quarter of those engaging in vaginal intercourse, and an eighth of those engaging in oral-genital sex. Thus, if people were engaging in high-risk behaviors with infected partners, most do not appear to be taking the precautions required to prevent HIV transmission. As described above, however, most people also report limiting their sexual activity to one partner. This will mitigate the spread of HIV, despite the infrequency of condom use. Those who believe themselves to be in mutually exclusive sexual partnerships may consider condoms unnecessary for prophylaxis.

The proportions engaging in various activities reported above overstate the occurrence of sexual activity among all county residents who are sexually active, because respondents who did not happen to be

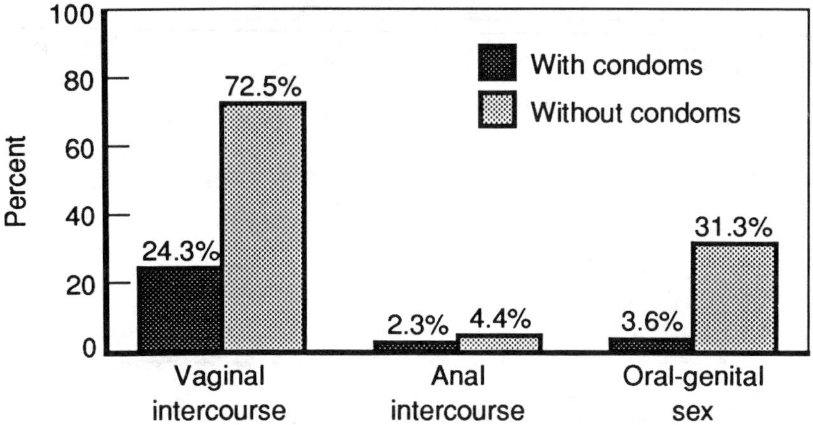

Fig. 2—Sexual practices in Los Angeles County among respondents sexually active in the past four weeks (n = 838)

sexually active during the four-week period are excluded. For a more general cross-sectional portrait of sexual activity in Los Angeles County, these respondents should be included, as they are in Fig. 3. Although the estimated proportions of people engaging in particular behaviors are lower when all residents are included, the relative frequencies of behavior are, of course, unchanged.

FREQUENCY OF SEXUAL PRACTICES BY TYPE OF RELATIONSHIP

Although gauging the proportion of the general public who engage in each type of sexual practice provides an important frame of reference, none of these sexual behaviors are practiced in isolation or performed in a mutually exclusive fashion. One respondent may engage in a variety of practices in a given four-week period. There is also an important distinction between being very sexually active and engaging in behaviors that are risky in terms of HIV transmission.

We therefore examined the mean frequency of each sexual practice in the context of different types of relationships, which provides a better context than behavior alone for assessing the extent to which respondents' activity was placing them at increased risk of HIV infection (Table 4). We examined the behavior within the following relationships: (1) married, (2) in an exclusive relationship with a primary partner, (3) in a nonexclusive relationship with a primary partner, (4)

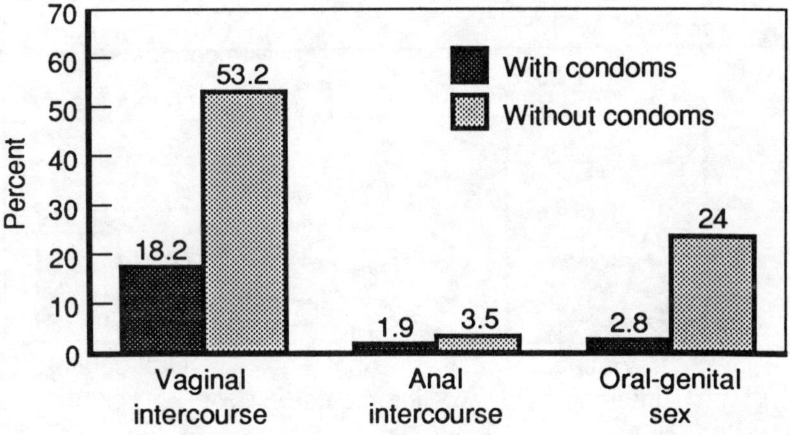

Fig. 3—Sexual practices among respondents sexually active in the past five years (n = 1,136) whether or not they reported a sexual partner in the past four weeks

neither married nor in another primary relationship, and (5) all other types of relationships (in this case, among same-sex relationships).[28]

Unprotected vaginal intercourse occurs, for the most part, in the context of being married or in other primary relationships, whether exclusive or not. Being in a primary relationship apparently confers the availability of a sexual partner that makes frequent sexual activity a possibility. At the same time, those without a primary partner report more than one sexual encounter on average in the past four weeks.

Condom use with vaginal intercourse is twice as frequent among those in nonexclusive relationships with a primary partner as among those in other types of relationships. Possibly those in "open" relationships have a heightened awareness of the need to take more precautions against disease while one is sexually active with more than one partner. However, it is equally plausible that those in nonexclusive relationships use condoms more frequently for contraceptive purposes. Our data do not allow us to determine with whom the condoms are being used, the "primary" partner or the additional partner(s) seen outside the relationship.

Surprisingly, respondents who report that they are not involved in a relationship with a primary partner are no more likely than others to use condoms more frequently for vaginal intercourse. Although they

[28]Relationships were categorized on the basis of type of relationship and gender match of partner. Too few of the respondents (n = 14) indicated same-sex relationships to enable us to characterize the frequency of sexual practices within parallel categories.

Table 4

MEAN FREQUENCY OF VAGINAL AND ANAL INTERCOURSE IN THE PAST FOUR WEEKS BY TYPE OF RELATIONSHIP

Type of Relationship	No. of Respondents	Total	With Condom	Without Condom
Vaginal				
Married (opposite sex)	520	5.3 (6.6)	0.7 (3.1)	4.6 (6.1)
In other primary relationship (opposite sex)				
Exclusive	186	7.0 (8.9)	1.7 (4.8)	5.3 (8.1)
Not exclusive	55	8.7 (7.9)	3.9 (7.2)	4.5 (5.5)
Neither married nor in other primary relationship (opposite sex)	176	1.6 (3.4)	0.8 (2.1)	0.9 (2.3)
All others[a]	14	3.8 (2.9)	2.0 (2.5)	0.9 (1.9)
Anal				
Married (opposite sex)	520	0.22 (1.37)	0.04 (0.44)	0.19 (1.25)
In other primary relationship (opposite sex)				
Exclusive	186	0.27 (1.27)	0.06 (0.53)	0.21 (1.15)
Not exclusive	55	0.51 (2.28)	0.44 (2.20)	0.07 (0.26)
Neither married nor in other primary relationship (opposite sex)	176	0.05 (0.23)	0.04 (0.21)	0.01 (0.09)
All others[a]	14	0.13 (0.58)	0.0 (0.0)	0.13 (0.58)

[a]Respondents in same-sex relationships. Respondents whose type of relationship was unknown were excluded.

are not as sexually active as those with established partners, they are engaging in unprotected sexual practices that place them at potential risk of HIV transmission.

Even though the practice of anal intercourse is relatively rare for the sample as a whole, we find similar patterns in the mean frequency of anal intercourse for each type of relationship, with the exception of those respondents who are in nonexclusive relationships with a primary partner.

Variables Associated with Practicing Unprotected Vaginal and Anal Intercourse

Among women in California, heterosexual contact is of roughly equal importance to IV drug use as a mode of HIV transmission (Capell and Schiller, 1990). This contrasts with the situation in most of the nation, where IV drug use is a more important mode. Given the frequency of unprotected sexual activity and its potential importance, we examined the predictors of engaging in unprotected vaginal and anal intercourse. We used a multiple regression model that included as predictor variables age, gender, race/ethnicity,[29] education,[30] household income,[31] employment status,[32] relationship status,[33] self-identification as

---

[29]Racial/ethnic categories were black, Hispanic, Asian, and a category "other" (which included respondents who did not report falling into one of the other categories), with whites as the omitted (comparison) category.

[30]Categorized as high school graduate, some college or more, and less than a high school diploma (omitted category).

[31]Based on a series of items asking whether the respondent's annual household income for 1988 was above or below a specified amount. Taken together, these items enabled us to determine a range within which each respondent's household income fell (e.g., $20,000 to $35,000). We estimated each respondent's household income at the midpoint of the range (e.g., $27,500), and assigned incomes of $100,000 or more the value of $100,000. Income distributions tend not to be symmetrical within ranges, so we would not recommend this procedure as a way to derive precise and unbiased population estimates of mean household income. It is a useful approximation, however, for purposes of evaluating the relationship of income to other variables. Household income was not measured for self-identified gay/bisexual men, so annual personal income for 1988 was used instead.

[32]Respondents were asked "Are you now: (1) working full-time, (2) working part-time, (3) with a job, but not at work because of illness, vacation, or strike, (4) unemployed, laid off, or looking for work, (5) retired, disabled, or no longer working, (6) in school, (7) keeping house, or (8) none of the above?" We compared those respondents who were employed full- or part-time to all other unemployed categories (3–8).

[33]Relationship status combined marital status, participation in another type of primary relationship, degree of exclusivity within a primary relationship, and gender of partner. We examined the contribution of being married to a member of the opposite sex and being in an exclusive primary relationship to other relationship types.

gay/bisexual,[34] knowing someone who has AIDS,[35] and AIDS-related knowledge (of both casual and noncasual modes of HIV transmission).

Predictors of Who Engages in Unprotected Anal Intercourse

Engaging in unprotected anal intercourse is quite risky if one partner is infected with HIV; the risk appears to be greatest if the uninfected partner is in the receptive role.

Although the occurrence of anal intercourse was concentrated in a small percentage of the sample,[36] the variables associated with engaging in unprotected anal intercourse (see Table A.1) were:

- Being male;
- Being married; and
- Being in an exclusive primary relationship.

Self-identifying as homosexual or bisexual also tended to be associated with this behavior, but perhaps because of the small sample size, the relationship was not statistically significant ($p = 0.097$). Respondents' widely held belief that they were in a sexually exclusive relationship may have contributed to their willingness to engage in this generally risky practice.

Since few of our male respondents reported male-to-male sex contact, most of the anal intercourse they reported was presumably with a female partner. Thus, one might expect that the total amount reported by male and female respondents would be about the same. Instead, a significantly larger number of males reported engaging in this practice. There are various possible reasons for this asymmetric result. First, we note that our respondents were sampled as individuals, not as couples, so that the men and women were reporting on parallel but not shared experiences. Selection effects might have operated somewhat differently for men and women in our sample,

---

[34]We sought to determine whether being self-identified as gay or bisexual has an independent effect that is not explained by other sociodemographic and relationship variables.

[35]Respondents were classified as to whether they knew one or more persons with AIDS (31 percent) or did not know anyone with AIDS (69 percent).

[36]When a logistic regression model is fitted within the area of the binomial curve near 0 or 1, as in the present case, the fit can produce anomalous results (predicted values outside the allowable range of 0 to 1). We fitted the model anyway, not to obtain a reasonable quantitative fit but to determine which characteristics are significantly associated with this potentially risky sexual practice. The estimated coefficients and their standard errors provide this information even where there may be problems with fitted values. However, because of those problems we caution against using the regression results in Table A.1 to make quantitative predictions regarding the proportions of people with particular characteristics who engage in this practice.

leading to a lower representation of women than of men who had recently engaged in this practice. Second, men may simply be more willing than women to report this practice.[37]

Two variables were significantly associated with *not* engaging in anal intercourse:

- Having at least some college education; and
- Having accurate information about the likelihood of acquiring HIV through casual sources.

Even though it is still not a frequent practice, respondents with less than a high school education engage in unprotected anal intercourse more frequently than do those with high school diplomas.[38] It is perhaps not surprising that those who knew more about AIDS and did not have misconceptions about the risks of casual contacts were less likely to engage in unprotected anal intercourse. Knowledge about transmission through casual contact had predictive value even when education and other demographic variables were controlled for, however. Blacks tended to be less likely than whites to engage in unprotected anal intercourse, but the difference was not statistically significant ($p = 0.076$).

Predictors of Unprotected Vaginal Intercourse

We also examined variables predicting the propensity to engage in unprotected vaginal intercourse. Like unprotected anal intercourse, unprotected vaginal intercourse becomes "risky" (in the sense considered here) only if practiced with a partner infected with HIV or with various other sexually transmitted pathogens.

We found several variables associated with the propensity to engage in unprotected vaginal intercourse, as measured by an indicator variable for having done so in the last four weeks (see Table A.2). They include:

---

[37]Kinsey et al. (1948) compared the reports of pairs of spouses on frequency and type of sexual activity. They found high agreement overall, but men were significantly more likely to report having "rear-entry" intercourse than were their wives (24.6 percent compared with 17.4 percent of 224 pairs of spouses). It is not known whether there is a similar difference in reporting by gender for anal intercourse.

[38]We examined mean frequency of unprotected anal intercourse among those with less than a high school education ($n = 161$) compared with those with a high school diploma or better ($n = 934$). We found nearly a threefold difference in the frequency with which the two groups engaged in unprotected anal intercourse (mean frequency = 0.37 for less than high school, 0.11 for high school or better, $t = 3.15$, d.f. = 1,093, $p < 0.002$).

- Being male;
- Being 25 to 34 years old or 45 to 54 years old;
- Being married (to someone of the opposite sex);
- Being in an exclusive primary relationship; and
- Having a high degree of knowledge regarding the likelihood of acquiring HIV through noncasual sources (e.g., sexual behavior, and sharing needles).

This model does not provide us with any substantive information that would help us draw conclusions about the risk inherent in practicing unprotected vaginal intercourse. It is the modal (most common) behavior in the general population and seems to occur most often among married men and women or within exclusive primary relationships. Almost all age groups engage in this form of sexual activity in roughly equivalent proportions, with some decreases in the number of people who engage in it after the age of 55 years.

Knowledge of noncasual modes of transmission is high and apparently has no influence on use of condoms during vaginal sex.

Frequency of Condom Use

In addition to asking about specific sexual practices with and without condoms, we also measured how often people reported using condoms overall. This is a broader measure of condom use in that we included responses from people who had not reported a sexual partner in the past four weeks.[39] Nearly 60 percent reported that they never used condoms, whereas less than 12 percent reported that they use them all of the time (Table 5).

To find out which respondent characteristics are associated with self-reported frequency of condom use, we used ordinary least squares (OLS) multiple regression to explore the relationship of frequency of use to a series of sociodemographic and AIDS-related variables, such as age, gender, race/ethnicity, and AIDS-related knowledge.[40]

We found several variables significantly associated with using condoms infrequently (see Table A.3):

---

[39]At the same time, it excluded those who reported no sexual partners in the past five or ten years.

[40]In this regression model, we assigned successive integer values to each of the response categories (e.g., 1 = "all of the time," 2 = "most of the time," and so on) and treated these values as a continuous (dependent) variable. Given this model specification, coefficients are in the direction of predicting infrequent condom use.

Table 5

PERCENTAGE DISTRIBUTION OF
RESPONDENTS' FREQUENCY
OF CONDOM USE

Frequency	Percentage
All of the time	12
Most of the time	7
A good bit of the time	3
Some of the time	8
A little of the time	13
None of the time	57

NOTE: Asked of 1,108 respondents who reported having been sexually active in the past five years, excluding 149 who have not been sexually active in the past five years, 37 who said that they do not currently have sex, nine who refused to answer the question, and two who did not know how often they use condoms.

- Being 35 years old or more;
- Being currently married; and
- Being in an exclusive primary relationship.

No other demographic features predicted condom use, nor did AIDS-related knowledge of noncasual modes of transmission (e.g., through sexual intercourse) have any apparent relationship to the frequency of condom use. As results presented below indicate, it seems likely that people in these groups generally do not regard themselves as being at risk for HIV transmission. So long as neither partner is infected and these relationships remain exclusive, there is no reason that they should.

WHY PEOPLE DO NOT USE CONDOMS

We asked respondents who did not use condoms all of the time their reasons for not using them. They were asked to rate each of a series of statements about why they did not use condoms (e.g., they are uncomfortable) on a five-point scale from definitely true to definitely false. Table 6 summarizes their responses.

The foremost reason for not using condoms is respondents' belief that neither they nor their partners are at risk for AIDS (78 percent rated this reason as definitely or mostly true). The types of

Table 6

PERCENTAGE DISTRIBUTION OF RESPONDENTS' REASONS FOR NOT USING CONDOMS

Reason	Definitely True	Mostly True	Equally True or False	Mostly False	Definitely False
My partner(s) and I are not at risk for AIDS	63	15	7	4	11
Sex is usually less enjoyable with a condom	28	20	13	12	28
When I'm high on alcohol or drugs, I don't think about it	12	7	8	8	66
Condoms are not easily available when I need one	11	6	11	11	61
Condoms break or leak	8	8	16	14	54
It's embarrassing to buy condoms	7	7	11	11	64
Not comfortable talking to my partner about them	7	6	11	14	63
Do not know how to use a condom properly	4	3	11	11	70
Condoms are too expensive	3	2	14	15	66

NOTE: Asked of 978 respondents who were sexually active in the past five years and reported that they used condoms less than "all of the time." Percentages excluded from 31 to 78 respondents (depending upon the reason) who refused to answer the question or did not know how to rate a particular reason.

relationships and degree of exclusivity reported by respondents suggest that only a small proportion may be at risk of HIV transmission through their sexual behavior, and some of these are among the nearly 12 percent who use condoms all the time. Insofar as these beliefs are accurate, efforts to increase the use of condoms could be tailored more efficiently to address the needs of those who are at higher risk of acquiring HIV infection (e.g., those not in exclusive primary relationships).

We have shown that condoms are used infrequently by those who are married or in other primary relationships that they report to be exclusive (Table A.3). We next examined how respondents' beliefs about their risk of getting AIDS vary with the type of relationship. As shown in Table 7, respondents who were married or in primary exclusive relationships (with the same or opposite sex) were more likely to see themselves as not being at risk for AIDS. However, two-thirds of those in nonexclusive relationships or those without a primary partner also saw themselves as not being at risk for AIDS.

Another significant percentage (48 percent) gave as a reason for not using condoms that condoms made sex less enjoyable. These findings parallel those found among gay/bisexual men in Los Angeles County (Kanouse et al., 1991), showing that some of the major barriers to condom use are similar among homosexuals and heterosexuals. Although the problems inherent in overcoming the "pleasure

Table 7

PERCEPTIONS OF NOT BEING AT RISK BY RELATIONSHIP STATUS AMONG RESPONDENTS NOT USING CONDOMS

Type of Relationship	No. of Respondents	Percentage Who Consider Self and Partner Not at Risk[a]
Married (opposite sex)	520	83
In other primary relationship (opposite sex)		
Exclusive	186	73
Not exclusive	55	66
Neither married nor in other primary relationship (opposite sex)	176	67
All others (same sex)[b]	14	73
All respondents	951	78

[a]Percentage of respondents who rate the statement "My partner and I are not at risk of AIDS" as "definitely" or "mostly" true. This statement was rated only by sexually active respondents who use condoms less than "all the time." The differences among the percentages shown in this table are statistically significant, chi square = 24.61, d.f. = 4, $p < 0.001$.

[b]Constituted remaining respondents in same-sex relationships. Other respondents whose type of relationship was unknown were excluded.

factor" have been met with some innovative programs designed to, for example, eroticize condom use in the gay community, so far as we know, little work has been done on ways to effectively overcome this particular barrier in heterosexuals.

Other reasons, such as forgetting to use a condom when "high," concerns about condoms breaking, not having one available when needed, and difficulties in buying or talking about condoms with a partner, have reduced condom use only for a small proportion of the public (less than 20 percent reporting "definitely" or "mostly true" for each of these reasons). Nonetheless, those who fail to use condoms for these reasons are potential targets for educational information aimed, for example, at helping people plan ahead to avoid being unprepared, or to negotiate condom use with a sexual partner.

PREVALENCE OF ALCOHOL AND DRUG USE IN LOS ANGELES COUNTY

Background

Use of alcohol and drugs is relevant to the spread of HIV infection for three reasons. First, the use of intravenous drugs (specifically, the sharing of infected needles or other drug paraphernalia) poses a substantial direct risk of HIV transmission. Second, in a growing number of reported AIDS cases the only risk behavior has been having sex with an intravenous drug user. Third, the use of alcohol or drugs in conjunction with sexual activity may be associated with practicing "unsafe" sex (Leigh, 1990; Minkoff et al., 1989; Siegel et al., 1989; Stall et al., 1986; Valdiserri et al., 1988).

Our goals in asking questions about alcohol and drug use were limited to providing a broad-based portrait of use in the general population in Los Angeles County. We tried to gauge the rough proportion of the general population who drink or use drugs, the frequency with which they do either, and the extent to which they use them in conjunction with sexual activity. We did not obtain sufficiently detailed information to permit a close examination of patterns of substance use, nor are we in a position to quantify the risk associated with these substance use estimates.

It is highly unlikely that a household-based telephone survey would capture such information from many of those who are most actively engaged in drug use, and undoubtedly, these results underestimate substance use in Los Angeles County. However, intravenous drug use has been less important as a risk factor for AIDS in Los

Angeles County than it has been in many other urban areas, so there is less reason here to focus on this topic.[41]

Alcohol Use

We asked respondents if they had ever drunk alcohol, and, if so, how often they had drunk in the past four weeks.[42] The vast majority of respondents said that they had drunk alcohol at least once before (87 percent). This is comparable to national population estimates based on the National Household Survey of Drug Abuse (National Institute on Drug Abuse, 1990). Table 8 shows the frequency with which people reported having drunk alcohol in the previous four weeks.

Table 8

PERCENTAGE DISTRIBUTION OF RESPONDENTS' ALCOHOL USE IN THE PAST FOUR WEEKS

Frequency	Percentage
Every day	3
Almost every day	4
3 to 4 days a week	7
1 to 2 days a week	21
Less than once a week	28
Not at all	37

NOTE: Asked of 1,140 respondents who said that they had drunk alcohol, excluding one respondent who refused to answer.

[41]The prevalence of HIV infection among intravenous drug users in Los Angeles County has recently been estimated to be no higher than 8 percent—considerably lower than in some East Coast cities (Longshore and Anglin, 1990). The reasons for the lower rate of infection in Los Angeles County probably have to do with regional differences in the social context of drug use (Watters, 1989); drug injectors on the West Coast are less likely to share injection equipment in ways that facilitate rapid transmission of HIV across social networks—for example, by sharing injection equipment with strangers or by frequenting large "shooting galleries" that serve 100 or more patrons daily. The risk behaviors that spread HIV do occur among Los Angeles County's intravenous drug users, however, and under the right conditions, seroprevalence rates could increase rapidly (Longshore and Anglin, 1990).

[42]The same rationale described for four-week recall periods for sexual behavior applies to questions posed for alcohol and drug use.

The majority have drunk very little or not at all in the past month (65 percent), although about one in five report drinking alcohol one to two days a week. Roughly 7 percent report drinking alcohol every day or almost every day, consistent with national data indicating that 7.5 percent of the total household population age 21 and older consumed alcohol on 20 or more days during the month preceding a 1988 interview (National Institute on Drug Abuse, 1990). The percentage reporting no alcohol use at all during the preceding four weeks is somewhat lower than the 45 percent of respondents aged 21 and over who reported no alcohol use in the preceding month (National Institute on Drug Abuse, 1990). Rates of use tend to be higher among residents of large metropolitan areas.

Nonmedical Drug Use in Los Angeles County

We asked all respondents whether they had ever used drugs such as marijuana, cocaine, amyl nitrates ("poppers"), amphetamines, tranquilizers, LSD, PCP, heroin, or other drugs for "recreational or nonmedical purposes." Thirty-one percent indicated that they had used drugs nonmedically at one time or another. For those with such a history, we asked about use of any of the same drugs in the past four weeks. Roughly one in five (18 percent) reported such recent drug use.[43]

Marijuana was by far the most popular nonmedical drug among recent users (90 percent), followed by cocaine (16 percent) (see Table 9). No other drugs were used by more than about 5 percent of recent drug users. On average, those who used marijuana did so nine times during the four weeks.

We also asked respondents who had ever used drugs whether they had ever used drugs intravenously or done skin popping, and, if so, how many times in the past 12 months (regardless of the kind of intravenous drug used). Five percent (or 1.6 percent of the total sample) indicated that they had tried intravenous drugs at least once before, with only 6 percent of that group having used intravenous drugs in the past year (this amounts to one person in the total sample). This is low in comparison to NIDA (1990) estimates of the prevalence of intravenous drug use in the population.

As we have noted, many active drug users may be outside established households, unavailable by telephone, and unwilling to disclose

[43]This refers to one in five of those asked the question, not of the entire general population sample. Therefore, 18 percent of the 31 percent (or less than 6 percent of the total sample) have recently used one or more of these drugs for a nonmedical purpose.

Table 9

PATTERNS OF RECENT DRUG USE AMONG DRUG USERS IN THE PAST FOUR WEEKS

Drugs Used Once or More	Percentage Using[a]	Percentage Using in Total Sample	Frequency of Use		
			No.	Mean	S.D.
Any drug	100	6	—	—	—
Marijuana or hashish	90	5	66	9.0	21.8
Crack	5	<1	3	2.2	1.9
Other forms of cocaine	16	<1	12	1.6	0.9
Amyl or butyl nitrates (poppers, rush, or snaps)	2	<1	1	12	—
Stimulants or uppers (amphetamines, speed, or crystal)	9	<1	5	2.0	1.3
Hallucinogens (MDA, LSD [acid], PCP, mescaline, ecstasy, or mushrooms)	4	<1	4	1.7	1.9
Tranquilizers, sedatives, pain killers, "downers"	7	<1	5	4.2	4.7
Opiates (heroin or morphine)	1	<1	1	2	—

[a]Only 6 percent of the total sample reported using one or more drugs for a recreational, nonmedical purpose in the past four weeks.

illegal behavior, making it difficult to capture information from them in a telephone survey. Even so, telephone surveys in areas that probably have more intravenous drug users than Los Angeles County have revealed somewhat larger numbers of them than we did.[44] Thus, one reason we may not have captured many in our survey may be that they are not as numerous in Los Angeles County as elsewhere.

[44]For example, Hingson et al. (1990) conducted a telephone survey of 1,323 Massachusetts residents selected using stratified random digit dialing. Thirty-three of their respondents (representing an estimated 1 percent of the statewide population) had used intravenous drugs in the last seven years.

How Often Do Sex and Drugs Mix?

The use of alcohol or drugs in conjunction with sexual activity may indirectly increase the risk of HIV transmission by lowering inhibitions and making people less cautious, although whether this is a major factor in the general population is unclear.[45] We asked all respondents who had ever consumed alcohol how often they drank it before or during sex in the previous 12 months. A parallel question was asked of all sexually active[46] respondents who reported that they had ever used drugs (31 percent of the sample, compared with the 6 percent who had used drugs in the past four weeks).

Table 10 shows the frequency with which alcohol or drugs were used in conjunction with sex.

Only 7 percent reported using alcohol at least "a good bit of the time" before or during sexual activity; another 13 percent used it some of the time. Over half reported that they never drank alcohol before or during sexual activity. About 9 percent of those who reported having ever tried drugs admitted to using drugs before or during sex at least some of the time.

These results do not show widespread use of alcohol or drugs in conjunction with sex, but there may be a small proportion of individuals in the general population whose sexual behavior (particularly preventive practices) may be affected by substance use.

KNOWLEDGE ABOUT AIDS

Increasing the public's knowledge about modes of HIV transmission has frequently been touted as the primary tool for preventing the spread of the epidemic from the major "risk groups" into the general population. Previous studies, such as the National Health Interview Survey's special supplement on AIDS-related knowledge and atti-

[45]Whether the "disinhibiting" effects of alcohol and drugs result in more frequent practicing of unsafe sex has been the focus of research among gay/bisexual men as investigators have explored the sociological factors that contribute to increased risk of HIV transmission. Although it is plausible that alcohol or drug use reduces the extent to which men and women take precautions, parallel studies aimed at gauging the effects of alcohol and drugs on subsequent risk of HIV infection or other sexually transmitted diseases have not to our knowledge been conducted on general population samples.

[46]We included anyone who had had at least one sexual partner in the past five years, except those respondents who indicated, when asked about alcohol use in conjunction with sexual activity, that they had not had sex in the past 12 months.

Table 10

PERCENTAGE DISTRIBUTION OF RESPONDENTS' ALCOHOL AND DRUG USE BEFORE OR DURING SEX IN THE PAST FOUR WEEKS

Frequency	Alcohol and Sex[a] (n = 981)	Drug and Sex[b] (n = 392)
All of the time	1	1
Most of the time	3	1
A good bit of the time	3	1
Some of the time	13	6
A little bit of the time	27	14
None of the time	54	77

[a]Excludes 63 respondents who reported not having sex in the past 12 months, nine who refused to answer the question, and one who did not know how frequently he/she had used alcohol before or during sex. Also excludes 79 respondents who were asked an earlier version of the question with different response categories.

[b]Excludes all respondents who reported never having tried drugs for a nonmedical purpose (69 percent of the sample). Also excludes one respondent who had tried drugs but was not sexually active in the past 12 months and one who refused to answer the question.

tudes[47] (Hardy, 1990a, 1990b) and the 1988 statewide survey sponsored by the California Department of Health Services Office of AIDS (Capell and Schiller, 1990; Capell et al., 1990),[48] have shown that most people can identify the groups at highest risk of HIV infection and the major modes of transmission (e.g., through sexual behavior or by sharing infected needles). At the same time, many people have major misconceptions about the likelihood of HIV transmission through casual contact (Kappel et al., 1989; Turner et al., 1989a).

---

[47]The National Health Interview Survey (NHIS) is a continuous cross-sectional probability sample of U.S. households that may be weighted to represent the total U.S. civilian noninstitutionalized population. Special supplements are included every year that cover a range of health-related topics. AIDS-related attitudes and knowledge have been surveyed in the most recent supplement, with preliminary results reported quarterly.

[48]The survey was conducted by Communication Technologies, Inc., the organization responsible for the conduct of five waves of the random digit dial (RDD) surveys in San Francisco. RDD methods were used to draw samples of the general population in proportion to the number of households in each geographic area of the state. The initial sample was augmented by additional RDD samples in areas with higher minority representation.

We examined several questions bearing on AIDS-related knowledge:

1. What is the level of knowledge among the general public in Los Angeles County regarding perceived and actual modes of HIV transmission?
2. What are the variables that predict high and low levels of AIDS-related knowledge? Are there subgroups in Los Angeles with gaps in their knowledge of AIDS that might be filled through additional education/prevention efforts?
3. To what extent is knowledge about AIDS associated with practicing fewer risky behaviors?

We asked all respondents about ways in which AIDS might be spread. For each item, we asked them to rate the likelihood on a scale from 1 ("very likely") to 4 ("very unlikely") that a person would get AIDS from a particular activity (e.g., living near a home or hospital for AIDS patients). Table 11 summarizes the responses to the individual items.

Almost universally, respondents correctly assessed the high risk of HIV transmission associated with sharing uncleaned needles with an infected intravenous drug user or with having unprotected sex with someone who is infected with HIV. They also understood the potential for perinatal transmission from an infected mother to her baby. The AIDS-related knowledge of many respondents extended little further than that, however.

Over 80 percent saw blood transfusions as "somewhat" to "very likely" to lead to infection with the AIDS virus. This response may reflect the general perception that the blood supply is not particularly safe.[49] However, it is also possible that respondents were registering their (correct) belief that if a unit of blood is contaminated, then transfusion is a highly efficient means of HIV transmission. However, this does not explain why 28 percent thought that *donating* blood poses a relatively high risk. People may tend to assume that the needles used in drawing blood are reused and hence pose a risk of transmission from one donor to the next.

About one in five believe that it is somewhat to very unlikely that a person could be infected with the AIDS virus and not have any symptoms. This reflects an important lack of understanding of carrier states and the likelihood that someone could carry the virus yet display no outward signs or symptoms for a long time.

---

[49]Thirty-eight percent of the total sample (n = 1,296, excluding nine respondents who said they did not know how they would rate the safety of the blood supply) regarded the blood supply as somewhat to very unsafe.

Table 11

PERCENTAGE DISTRIBUTION OF RESPONDENTS' KNOWLEDGE ABOUT HIV TRANSMISSION

Mode of Transmission	Very Likely	Somewhat Likely	Somewhat Unlikely	Very Unlikely
From sharing uncleaned needles for drug use with someone who has the AIDS virus	95	3	1	2
Any person with the AIDS virus can pass it on to someone else through sexual intercourse without a condom	92	5	1	1
A pregnant woman who has the AIDS virus can pass it on to her baby	91	7	0	2
From getting a blood transfusion	60	21	12	7
From donating blood	16	12	16	55
From eating in a restaurant whose cook has the AIDS virus	15	27	28	30
From being bitten by a mosquito	13	26	21	40
From using public toilets	11	18	21	50
From being around someone with AIDS who is coughing or sneezing	8	25	28	40
From attending school with a child who has the AIDS virus	6	15	25	54
From living near a home or hospital for AIDS patients	6	11	16	68
A person can be infected with the AIDS virus and not have symptoms of AIDS	54	27	13	7

NOTE: Asked of all 1,305 respondents. Number responding to each item varies slightly. Percentages do not all sum to 100 on account of rounding.

Clearly, there is substantial confusion or misperception of the likelihood of transmission of the AIDS virus through casual contact. Over 40 percent believe that it is somewhat to very likely that one could get AIDS from eating in a restaurant where the cook has AIDS. Nearly 40 percent have similar beliefs about the probability of getting infected from a mosquito bite. Roughly equivalent proportions (about 30 percent each) regard it as somewhat to very likely that a person can become infected with HIV simply by being around someone with AIDS who is coughing or sneezing, or by using public toilets.

Six of the survey items concerned with AIDS/HIV transmission by casual contact were identical or nearly identical to items employed in the National Health Interview Survey AIDS Supplement (Hardy, 1990b), administered to a national sample of 40,689 persons 18 years of age and older who were interviewed between January and December 1989. Across these six items, 47 percent of Los Angeles County residents gave the correct answer, compared with 59 percent in the nationally representative sample surveyed the same year (Hardy, 1990b).[50] Thus, misperceptions about transmission through casual contact appear to be more common among Los Angeles County residents than among U.S. residents as a whole. In part, this may reflect the county's demographic composition, with a high concentration of racial and ethnic populations that suffer from knowledge gaps with respect to HIV transmission through casual contact (see the discussion below).

These findings indicate that although most people are aware of the ways in which the AIDS virus is transmitted, many have still not distinguished these transmission modes from those that pose little or no risk. Misperception of the risks from casual contact with people who have AIDS could lead to unnecessary worry and, more seriously, could exacerbate unwarranted fears of and possible discrimination against people with AIDS and members of the risk groups that have been associated with the AIDS epidemic.

We also examined the social and demographic predictors of AIDS-related knowledge, performing OLS multiple regression analyses on two measures of knowledge constructed from the 12 items in Table

---

[50]The national sample scored higher on all six items: 49 percent compared with 30 percent for an item on eating in a restaurant; 43 compared with 40 percent for an item on mosquito bites; 60 compared with 50 percent for an item on using public toilets; 45 compared with 40 percent for an item on exposure to coughing or sneezing; 76 percent compared with 54 percent for an item on attending school with an infected child; and 83 percent compared with 68 percent for an item on living near a home or hospital for AIDS patients.

10:[51] (1) a three-item measure of knowledge about noncasual modes of HIV transmission,[52] and (2) an eight-item measure of knowledge about casual transmission or about ways in which the virus is not transmitted.[53] Items used in both measures were recoded as necessary so that a high knowledge score corresponded with a high level of AIDS-related knowledge. To facilitate interpretation and comparison across the groups, the two knowledge scores were then scaled to fall between 0 and 100 points.

The mean scale scores for all respondents were 96.5 for knowledge of noncasual modes of transmission and 64.7 for knowledge of the risks of transmission from casual contact. Several variables were associated with knowledge of the major modes of HIV transmission (see Table A.4):

- Being 35–44 years old;
- Having a high school diploma; and
- Having at least some college.

Our model predicting knowledge of the risks of casual contact generally explained more of the variation in scores across different sociodemographic groups than did our model of knowledge of noncasual modes of transmission.[54] Indeed, we found that most of the sociodemographic variables were significantly associated with knowledge of casual transmission in one way or another (see Table A.4). Variables associated with misperception of the risks associated with casual contact were:

---

[51]We used only 11 of the 12 items in constructing the knowledge scores. We excluded a question about the likelihood of getting infected through blood transfusions, since we had no way of determining whether respondents interpreted the question as conditional or unconditional on receiving an infected unit. (The likelihood of receiving an infected unit of blood is very low, but the likelihood of transmission if one does receive such a unit is very high.) The 11 items we included present no major ambiguities of interpretation and address topics for which clear epidemiological evidence is available.

[52]This measure included items on the sharing of needles or having sex with someone who is infected with the AIDS virus, as well as an item about perinatal transmission from an infected mother to her baby (Table 11).

[53]The measure of "knowledge about casual transmission" excluded the three noncasual items and the question about blood transfusions; it included an item measuring the respondent's assessment of the likelihood that someone infected with the AIDS virus may not exhibit symptoms, which does not concern transmission.

[54]The R^2 was 0.21052 compared with 0.041.

- Being 45 to 55 years old;
- Being nonwhite; and
- Being married.

All nonwhite racial/ethnic groups (black, Hispanic, Asian, or in another racial/ethnic category other than white) had disproportionately lower knowledge scores for risks associated with transmission from casual sources (Table 12). There were no significant differences in knowledge by gender.

Several variables were significantly associated with more accurate ratings of the likelihood of acquiring HIV infection through casual contact:

- Being a high school graduate;
- Having some college education;
- Having higher household income; and
- Knowing someone who has AIDS.

In contrast to the finding that married people are particularly misinformed about the risks of casual contact, people in exclusive unmarried primary relationships tend to be better informed about these risks ($p = 0.051$).

It is not surprising that education is associated with greater knowledge of the lack of risk associated with casual contact, but we cannot apply this finding as an evaluation of current educational efforts. The age range of our sample is such that most of our respondents graduated from school years ago. Moreover, those with more education tend to be exposed to more information and to comprehend and remember it better both while they are in school and later. Education and income are usually highly correlated, so the relationship with income is also understandable.

It has been speculated that as more people know someone who has been diagnosed with AIDS, knowledge related to AIDS risk will increase as people seek to clarify the risks surrounding transmission through casual contact or as they obtain information directly from friends, family, or people with AIDS. By this reasoning, it makes sense that people who already know someone who has been diagnosed with AIDS are significantly more likely to understand that casual contact poses little risk of transmission.

Table 12

PERCENTAGE DISTRIBUTION OF RESPONDENTS' KNOWLEDGE OF CASUAL AND NONCASUAL MODES OF TRANSMISSION BY DEMOGRAPHIC CHARACTERISTICS

Demographic Variables	Knowledge of Casual Modes Mean (S.D.)	Knowledge of Noncasual Modes Mean (S.D.)
Race/ethnicity		
White	73 (19)	98 (8)
Black	56 (14)	98 (4)
Hispanic	57 (26)	95 (18)
Asian	57 (26)	96 (16)
Other	61 (19)	99 (6)
Education		
< High school	51 (25)	92 (22)
High school graduate	64 (18)	97 (10)
> High school	69 (21)	98 (8)
Marital status		
Married	64 (24)	97 (11)
Divorced	65 (18)	97 (9)
Separated	61 (17)	97 (7)
Widowed	64 (17)	98 (6)
Never married/single	67 (21)	95 (15)
In a primary relationship		
Exclusive	66 (22)	97 (10)
Not exclusive	56 (23)	96 (8)

Relationship Between Knowledge and Behavior

We planned in our analyses to examine the links between knowledge of the major modes of transmission and the propensity to engage in risky behavior. If our analyses identify people who remain uninformed about the major modes of transmission and who also engage in behavior that places them at risk of HIV infection, this would suggest a potentially important role in primary prevention for targeted educational outreach efforts emphasizing the basic facts of transmission.

As it turns out, our results do not allow us to identify such a link; instead, we find that the majority of the public is aware of the basic modes of transmission and does not currently have sex with multiple partners or engage in unprotected anal intercourse. The absence of much variability in our measures of basic knowledge on the one hand

and risky sexual behavior or IV drug use on the other virtually precludes finding a relationship between the two, and indeed, we found none.

This does not necessarily mean that knowledge and behavior are unrelated for all subpopulations within the county. A survey focusing on a high-risk subpopulation might find such a link within that particular group. But for county residents as a whole, we believe that the results indicate that ignorance of the basic facts of transmission is no longer (if it ever was) the major barrier to behavior change for those currently engaging in risky behavior. We discuss this issue further in presenting our conclusions.

Perceived Effectiveness of Various Prevention Measures

Respondents were asked to rate the effectiveness of four methods that some people use to avoid getting AIDS through sexual activity: condoms, spermicidal agents alone, spermicidal agents with a diaphragm, and monogamous sex between two HIV-negative individuals (Table 13). Their assessment of the effectiveness of preventing HIV infection was rated highest for monogamous sex between two

Table 13

PERCENTAGE DISTRIBUTION OF RESPONDENTS' PERCEPTIONS OF DIFFERENT PREVENTION ACTIVITIES' EFFECTIVENESS

Prevention Activity	Very Effective	Somewhat Effective	Not at All Effective	Don't Know
Two people who do not have the AIDS virus having sex only with each other	73	14	12	1
Using a condom	42	50	7	1
Using a diaphragm with spermicidal cream or jelly	9	35	50	6
Using a spermicidal jelly, foam, or cream that contains non-oxynol-9 (that is, a spermicide alone without a condom or diaphragm)	7	32	53	8

NOTE: Asked of 1,136 respondents who reported having been sexually active in the past five years. Percentages exclude nine to 86 respondents who did not know how to rate the effectiveness of some of these activities.

HIV-negative people, although 12 percent felt that even in these circumstances, there were no assurances of safety from getting AIDS this way. Condom use, despite reported problems with breakage, leakage, and misuse, was rated as very effective by 42 percent of the respondents and as somewhat effective by another 50 percent. Respondents were much less certain about the effectiveness of spermicidal agents, regardless of whether they were used in conjunction with an alternative barrier method, such as the diaphragm.

SOURCES OF INFORMATION ABOUT AIDS

Exposure to information about AIDS can be important not only in conveying basic facts about transmission and methods of prevention but also in maintaining public awareness of AIDS as a preventable disease. Because AIDS-related knowledge and awareness are likely to have an important bearing on preventive behaviors and public response to the epidemic, it is important to determine how various segments of the public obtain information and what sources they find most trustworthy.

Respondents were asked about where they received most of their information about AIDS. Up to three mentions were recorded. As summarized in Table 14, nearly three-quarters of the respondents said that they received most of their AIDS information through television or radio, with magazines and newspapers being mentioned second most often (by 60 percent of the respondents). Brochures and pamphlets about AIDS from local, state, or federal agencies were mentioned by 25 percent of all respondents, followed by medical sources (17 percent mentioned doctors, hospitals, medical journals, or the American Red Cross). Other sources, such as AIDS hotlines, public lectures, school, friends/relatives, or churches, were also mentioned, but none of the individual categories were cited by more than about 15 percent of respondents.

Respondents were then asked to identify the most trustworthy source of information about AIDS that they used (also shown in Table 14). Nearly half trusted the information they obtained through medical sources the most, in contrast to what they reported using as their major sources of information. Only about one in five respondents reported that TV/radio was the most trustworthy source of AIDS information, although nearly three-quarters used this source.

For the county to plan effective information campaigns that address the needs of the diverse communities and groups within the county, it is important to determine the characteristics of the

Table 14

PERCENTAGE DISTRIBUTION OF RESPONDENTS' KNOWLEDGE OF INFORMATION SOURCES ABOUT AIDS

Source	Any Mention[a]	Single Most Trustworthy Mention
TV/radio	73	19
Magazines/newspapers	59	7
Brochures/pamphlets	25	16
Doctors/hospitals[b]	17	48
Other[c]	34	10

[a]Sums to more than 100 percent because more than one mention was allowed.

[b]Includes doctors, hospitals, medical journals, or the American Red Cross.

[c]Includes hotline, church, schools, public lectures, and friends/relatives, no single category of which represented more than 15 percent of all respondents.

audiences for each of the major information sources. High-risk behavior does not occur with equal frequency in all segments of the population but appears to concentrate in certain subgroups, suggesting the need to provide targeted education/prevention programs to the types of people most likely to engage in such behavior.[55] With that in mind, we examined the demographic and relationship variables that predict self-reported use of various sources of information about AIDS. We restricted our analysis to those sources mentioned by a sufficiently large number of respondents to enable us to conduct multivariate analyses.

We employed multiple logistic regression to determine the predictive value of variables such as age, race/ethnicity, and type of relationship (e.g., being in a primary nonexclusive relationship) in explaining respondents' mention of TV/radio (n = 833), magazines/newspapers (n = 675), pamphlets/brochures (n = 298), school (n = 121), friends/relatives (n = 170), and medical sources (n = 197) as the major source of AIDS information (Tables A.5 to A.10). Table 15 summarizes the results of these regressions by identifying the variables positively and negatively associated with mentioning each major information source.

[55]Even if the occurrence of risk behaviors were not concentrated, there are other reasons to consider a segmented targeting strategy as the most effective way to reach diverse subpopulations.

Table 15

DEMOGRAPHIC AND RELATIONSHIP VARIABLES THAT PREDICT MENTION OF MAJOR INFORMATION SOURCES

Source	No.	Variables Positively Associated with Mention	Variables Negatively Associated with Mention
TV/radio	833	Being 25–34 years old[a] Being 45–54 years old	Household income Being in a primary exclusive relationship
Magazines/ newspapers	675	Being 35–44 years old Being 45–54 years old Being 55–64 years old Being 65+ years old Some college education	Being black Being in a primary exclusive relationship[b]
Pamphlets/ brochures	298	Being black Being Hispanic	Being 45–54 years old Being 65+ years old
School	121	Some college education Being in a primary exclusive relationship Being in a primary open relationship[c]	Being 25–34 years old[a] Being 35–44 years old Being 45–54 years old Being 55–64 years old Being 65+ years old
Friends/ relatives	170	Being in a primary open relationship[d]	High school graduate Some college education
Medical sources	197	Being 25–34 years old[a,e] Being 35–44 years old Being 45–54 years old Being 55–64 years old	

[a]Each older age group is compared with 18- to 24-year-old respondents. This has particular significance for school as an information source, in that all age groups older than 25 are significantly less likely to obtain AIDS information from school or college.

[b]Of borderline significance at p = 0.053.

[c]Means do not differ significantly, but the p approaches a conventional level of significance (p = 0.052).

[d]Means do not differ significantly, but the p approaches a conventional level of significance (p = 0.059).

[e]Each age category differs from the 18- to 24-year-old age category with a probability that approaches but does not reach a conventional level of statistical significance (p = 0.059 to p = 0.062).

These findings suggest several targeting options:

- Targeting the key subgroup of 18- to 24-year-olds may best be achieved by channeling AIDS information through schools or colleges, beginning at younger ages to reach those who do not continue in school. This group also tends to rely more heavily than others on information from friends and relatives, which suggests the potential usefulness of outreach and education programs for peer students and parents.
- Blacks and Hispanics mention the use of AIDS pamphlets and brochures significantly more often than do whites and, on the average, do not cite magazines and newspapers as the source of most of their AIDS information.
- Other results suggest that those in primary open (nonexclusive) relationships rely on friends/relatives and school more than, for example, mass media for their AIDS information.[56] People in nonexclusive primary relationships are of various ages, and a targeted school or college-based approach may reach only the younger ones. For those who are older, campaigns focusing on locations for social gathering (e.g., bars or athletic events) might be worth considering.

PERCEIVED RISK OF ACQUIRING HIV INFECTION

We asked all respondents who reported being sexually active in the past five years (n = 1,156) to rate each of ten different sexual practices in terms of the risk of spreading AIDS, on a scale from 1 (not at all risky) to 10 (very risky).

These ratings can be taken as an indirect measure of knowledge, in that respondents' ratings can be compared to the relative risks for many of these practices suggested by epidemiological evidence. Although the true risks are not precisely known, the relative risks assigned to different behaviors by the public are of interest because they may suggest areas in which people consider it most necessary to be cautious in their personal behavior.

The behaviors perceived by the general public (Table 16) to be the most risky[57] were:

---

[56]Such individuals may spend more time interacting with people and less time attending to media.

[57]Defined as the behaviors rated as very risky (a score of 10) most often.

Table 16

PERCEIVED RISK OF SELECTED SEXUAL BEHAVIORS

Behaviors[a]	Mean	S.D.	Percentage Reporting Behavior as Very Risky[a]
Having sex without a condom with men who have sex with other men[b]	9.8	0.9	89
Having sex without a condom with a prostitute, either male or female	9.6	1.2	80
Having sex without a condom with many different partners	9.3	1.8	78
Having anal intercourse without a condom	9.1	1.8	68
Having vaginal intercourse without a condom	7.9	2.6	50
Having oral sex without a condom	7.5	2.9	45
Drinking alcohol or using drugs before or during sex	6.1	3.3	24
Having anal intercourse with a condom	5.2	3.1	16
Having oral sex with a condom	3.9	3.0	9
Having vaginal intercourse with a condom	3.7	2.7	4

[a]Perceived risk was rated on a scale from 1 (not at all risky) to 10 (very risky) for each type of sexual behavior or encounter. Excludes self-identified gay/bisexual respondents for whom the parallel battery did not permit melding of scores with the remainder of the general population sample.

[b]Asked of female respondents only for the subset of self-identified gay/bisexual men who were a part of the general population sample.

- Having sex without a condom with men who have sex with other men;[58]
- Having sex without a condom with a prostitute, either male or female;
- Having sex without a condom with many different partners; and,
- Having anal intercourse without a condom.

The perceived risk of unprotected vaginal intercourse was also relatively high (mean risk score of 8 on the 10-point scale), with respondents rating it as only slightly more risky than unprotected oral sex. Drinking alcohol or using drugs before or during sexual activity was also rated as a practice that has a higher-than-average risk of spreading HIV infection.

Activities perceived as presenting a low risk for spreading AIDS included having vaginal or oral-genital sex with condoms. Respondents considered having anal intercourse, even with a condom, as more risky than other sexual practices.

These results are consistent with our findings that the public is generally quite knowledgeable about the primary sexual modes of HIV transmission. However, taken alone, they do not provide any evidence about the degree to which perceived risk is related to personal behavior. Judgments about the risk of a behavior taken out of context may be accurate enough, but may not be seen as applying to the respondent or within the respondent's social network. Moreover, people may adjust their risk perceptions to justify their behavior or, alternatively, may choose their behaviors based on their risk perceptions. The data gathered in this survey provide no way for us to determine which of these processes is more important.

PERCEPTION OF THE RISK OF AIDS TO HEALTH CARE WORKERS

We asked all respondents (n = 1,305) to rate, on a scale from 1 (not at all risky) to 10 (very risky), how risky they thought taking care of people with AIDS is for different types of health care workers. Respondents were asked to make their ratings assuming that health care workers use the protective equipment available to them.

The risks to health care workers were almost uniformly rated as being only slightly above average (between a 5 or 6 on the 1–10 scale), and only 13 to 18 percent of the respondents rated any of these

[58]Asked of female respondents only.

occupations as being very risky (a score of 10) (Table 17). These ratings were lower than we expected in view of the much publicized, though relatively rare, incidents of health care workers' acquiring HIV infection from patients.

SELF-REPORTED BEHAVIOR CHANGE

In view of what is known about the risk behaviors related to HIV transmission, risk-reducing behavior change is the outcome sought by most education/prevention programs (Kelly et al., 1989; Joseph et al., 1987; Becker and Joseph, 1988). Although there is evidence that substantial changes have been made among gay and bisexual men, we know very little about how the AIDS epidemic has affected the behavior of others in the general population. Moreover, even when they occur, such changes may be difficult to sustain (Edgar et al., 1989; Stall et al., 1990).

Respondents' own global reports of having changed their behavior must be interpreted with caution. Both the ability and the motivation to accurately report changes in behavior over time are subject to

Table 17

PERCEIVED RISK OF AIDS TO HEALTH CARE WORKERS

Type of Health Care Workers	Mean[a]	S.D.	Percentage Reporting Job as Very Risky[a]
Physicians performing surgery on people with AIDS	5.7	3.0	18
Emergency room staff taking care of people with AIDS	5.8	3.0	17
Paramedics, firemen, and police dealing with people with AIDS	5.8	3.0	15
Home health care workers taking care of people with AIDS	5.0	3.0	13

[a]Perceived risk was rated on a scale from 1 (not at all risky) to 10 (very risky) for those health care workers described above. The percentage reporting the job as very risky is therefore the percentage rating the risk related to the job as a 10.

various errors and biases that limit the usefulness of the information provided.[59] Although many of these limitations are inherent in all types of surveys and study designs, they are particularly problematic in a cross-sectional survey such as ours. Nevertheless, such self-reports may provide a general indication of the types of changes that may have occurred in the general public and the degree to which those who have made them attribute these changes to the AIDS epidemic.

We asked respondents who had been sexually active in the last ten years (n = 1,180) to tell us whether they had made any changes in their social lives or sexual behavior because of AIDS. If, in their opinion, they had made one or more changes because of AIDS, they were then asked a series of questions about the specific changes they had made. For each change, we asked whether the reason for change was because of AIDS, for some other reason, or because of both AIDS and some other reason.

Table 18 summarizes the results. Only three of every ten respondents reported having made one or more lifestyle changes in response to the AIDS epidemic. This is in contrast to nearly nine out of every ten respondents in the parallel survey among gay and bisexual men (Kanouse et al., 1991). Most who reported changes said they had become more selective in choosing possible sexual partners, reduced the number of sexual partners (overall), and reduced the number of casual sexual partners. Sixty percent indicated that they had started to use condoms more often. Eighty to 90 percent of these specific changes were attributed to AIDS in whole or in part.

About 10 percent of the total sample said that they had stopped having anal intercourse. Similarly, nearly 10 percent of the male respondents (n = 78) said that they stopped having sex with prostitutes or hustlers. Finally, nearly half of the respondents who reported making changes reported lowering their alcohol or drug use, although most of this was attributed to reasons other than AIDS.

PUBLIC OPINION ABOUT AIDS

We asked all respondents a series of questions designed to elicit their general impressions of the epidemic and their opinions about several pertinent AIDS prevention policies. Public support, or the

[59]For example, respondents may report changes that they believe are socially desirable (e.g., match the presumed concerns of the researchers, agency, or interviewer). They may also fail to recall the nature or magnitude of changes accurately and may sincerely believe that they have made changes that they have not in fact made.

Table 18

PERCENTAGE DISTRIBUTION OF RESPONDENTS' REASONS FOR BEHAVIOR CHANGE[a]

Reported Change	Percentage Reporting This Change[b]	Because of AIDS	AIDS and Some Other Reason	Some Other Reason
Any change	29	29	—	—
Became celibate	3	48	38	14
Reduced number of sexual partners	21	44	46	10
Became more selective in choosing possible sexual partners	24	52	37	11
Reduced number of casual sexual partners	21	53	34	13
Started using condoms more often	16	56	24	20
Stopped having anal intercourse	9	52	37	11
Stopped having sex with prostitutes or hustlers[c]	8	60	28	12
Lowered alcohol or drug use	13	11	15	74

[a]Among those reporting making each change (sums to 100 percent).
[b]In total sample (excludes those not sexually active for ten years who were not eligible to make the changes by virtue of their inactivity).
[c]Asked of male respondents only.

lack thereof, has important implications for policymakers, legislators, and public health officials in Los Angeles County for programs that are supported by taxpayer dollars.

Even though most people are at little risk of acquiring HIV infection, it is clear that the AIDS epidemic has had an impact on how Los Angeles County residents conduct themselves and on how they think about risks to themselves and to others. We examined several indicators of the degree to which the epidemic has touched the lives of county residents.

Concern About AIDS

We asked all respondents to rate their general concern about AIDS on a scale from 1 (not concerned at all) to 10 (extremely concerned). About a third reported that they were extremely concerned about AIDS, giving the maximum possible value of 10 (Table 19).

The average rating was 7.5, suggesting that the majority of county residents view AIDS with great concern. At the same time, about one of every nine county residents reports not being at all concerned about AIDS.

Knowing People at Risk

To determine what proportion of the general public knew someone who was in a high risk category, respondents were read the following statement: "Some people have been found to be at higher risk for AIDS, like gay and bisexual men and intravenous drug users. Do you know anyone (either personally or professionally) who uses intravenous drugs?" This question was asked of respondents who were married or in other primary relationships, thereby excluding most self-identified gay/bisexual men, whose responses would inflate the estimated proportion of the general public knowing someone who was gay/bisexual.

Almost half (46 percent) the respondents reported that they knew at least one person who was homosexual or bisexual; 14 percent of the respondents indicated that they knew someone who was an intravenous drug user. We have no way to gauge the accuracy of these perceptions, but if they are accurate, it suggests that many county residents know someone who has an elevated risk of acquiring HIV infection.

Table 19

PERCENTAGE DISTRIBUTION OF RESPONDENTS' RATING OF CONCERN ABOUT AIDS

Rating	Percentage
10	33.7
8–9	28.2
6–7	13.5
4–5	13.4
1–3	11.2

NOTE: Asked of 1,305 respondents.

Knowing Someone with AIDS

All respondents were asked about the number of individuals whom they personally knew who had AIDS. Nearly one-third (31 percent) of all respondents knew at least one person with AIDS, living or dead (Table 20). This percentage may seem high considering the number of AIDS cases as a proportion of the total population of the county. At the same time, it is not far below the proportion of people who know someone in a high-risk category. If willingness to participate in the survey were related to concern about AIDS, respondents might have been somewhat more likely than most county residents to know both people with AIDS and people categorized as high-risk.

The majority of people with AIDS known by respondents were friends or acquaintances (66 percent among those knowing one person and 65 percent among those knowing two or more people with AIDS). At the same time, a substantial proportion were relatives,[60] coworkers, and patients or clients (Table 21).

Beliefs About the AIDS Epidemic

We asked respondents to indicate the extent of their agreement with statements made about the future magnitude of the AIDS epidemic,[61] about whether or not the news media are artificially inflating concern about AIDS,[62] and about willingness to work with someone who has AIDS or is HIV-infected.[63] Over 80 percent agree that AIDS will be a bigger problem in ten years; a similar percentage said they disagreed that the news media are distorting the public's view of the epidemic (Table 22).

Many respondents expressed discomfort with the idea of working in the same office with someone who is HIV-infected or has AIDS. Although slightly over 50 percent disagreed, our results indicate that about 25 percent of the public is somewhat to strongly resistant to the idea of working with people with AIDS or anyone who is HIV-

---

[60]This included relatives such as aunts, uncles, and cousins as well as parents, siblings, and children.

[61]Respondents were asked to indicate their agreement to the statement that "in ten years, AIDS will be a bigger problem than it is now" on a five-point scale from 1 (strongly agree) to 5 (strongly disagree).

[62]Respondents were asked to indicate their agreement to the statement that "AIDS is not as big a problem as the news media makes it out to be" on the same five-point scale.

[63]"I would not want to work in the same office as someone who has AIDS or is infected with the AIDS virus."

Table 20

NUMBER OF PEOPLE WITH AIDS RESPONDENTS KNOW PERSONALLY

Number Known[a]	No. of Respondents	Weighted Percentage
None	862	69
One	182	13
Two	107	8
Three or more	153	10

[a]Respondents were asked "How many people have you known personally, either living or dead, who came down with the AIDS virus?" The range of responses was from 0 to 500.

Table 21

RESPONDENTS' RELATIONSHIPS TO PEOPLE PERSONALLY KNOWN WITH AIDS

Relationship	Percentage Knowing One Person with AIDS[a] (n = 166)	Percentage Knowing Two or More Persons with AIDS[b] (n = 242)
Friend	39	46
Acquaintance	27	20
Coworker	14	19
Relative	11	6
Neighbor	5	4
Patient or client	4	5

[a]Those knowing one person with AIDS were asked "What (is/was) your relationship to that person?"

[b]Those knowing more than one person with AIDS were asked "What (is/was) your relationship to the person you (are/were) closest to?" Excludes 17 respondents who cited a relationship not covered by the categories provided or who refused to answer the question.

Table 22

PERCENTAGE DISTRIBUTION OF RESPONDENTS' OPINIONS ABOUT AIDS

Statement	Strongly Agree	Somewhat Agree	Are Neutral	Somewhat Disagree	Strongly Disagree
It is important for students in junior high and high school to be taught about AIDS prevention in school	94	4	1	1	0
It is important for students in elementary school to be taught about AIDS prevention in school	60	27	5	6	3
Public health officials should get the names of the sexual partners of people who have tested positive for the AIDS virus so they can be traced and notified[a]	68	15	7	4	6
In ten years, AIDS will be a bigger problem than it is now	63	20	9	6	3
I would not want to work in the same office as someone who has AIDS or is infected with the AIDS virus	12	12	25	19	32
AIDS is not as big a problem as the news media makes it out to be	9	8	6	20	58

[a]Asked of all respondents (n = 1,305) with the exception of the subset of self-identified gay/bisexual men who followed a skip logic through the summary that was parallel to the series used for the comparison survey among gay/bisexual men (Kanouse et al., 1991).

infected. This is consistent with the widespread misperceptions of the risk of casual contact with someone who is infected or has AIDS.

We examined the role that misperception of the risk of casual contact may play in this attitude toward people with AIDS by conducting an ordinary least squares (OLS) regression predicting the willingness to work with someone with AIDS. We included demographic variables, such as age, race/ethnicity, and education, and the summary knowledge score reflecting the risks of acquiring AIDS through casual contact.[64]

We found a strong relationship between misperception of the risks of casual contact and the willingness to work with someone with AIDS. The relationship was quite strong even after demographic factors had been controlled for (see Table A.11). This extends the findings of an earlier study by Stipp and Kerr (1989) of a relationship between education and willingness to have personal contact with people with AIDS.[65]

Public Opinion About AIDS Education/Prevention Activities

Although much of the cost of the AIDS epidemic is being paid for by public funds, little is known of the general public's views regarding the importance of different AIDS education/prevention policies, which programs they perceive to be most effective, and what their funding priorities would be.

AIDS Prevention Policies. We asked all respondents to indicate, on a five-point scale from 1 (strongly agree) to 5 (strongly disagree), the extent to which they agreed with several AIDS education/ prevention policies. These included (Table 22):

- AIDS education/prevention among junior high and high school students;
- AIDS education/prevention among elementary school students; and,
- Contact tracing and HIV partner notification.

---

[64]This score (described above), is a continuous measure of knowledge using eight items regarding the risk of acquiring HIV infection or AIDS through a variety of casual contact sources (e.g., from using a public toilet). A high score on the summary measure refers to a high degree of knowledge, in this case a perception of the risk of casual contact as being "not at all likely."

[65]Stipp and Kerr interpreted education as a proxy for exposure to information about AIDS, which was not directly measured in their study. Multivariate results of our study, in which knowledge and education are measured separately, indicate that knowledge is more strongly related than education to willingness to work with someone with AIDS, supporting Stipp and Kerr's interpretation.

There is substantial public support for AIDS prevention education to be taught at all school levels; 98 percent agree that such education is important for students in junior high and high school and 87 percent agree that it is important for students in elementary school. This finding sharply contrasts with the legislative and funding decisions made in Los Angeles County and the State of California.

Our survey also indicates broad support for contact tracing and partner notification of the sexual partners of people who have tested positive for the AIDS virus. Over two-thirds strongly agree with the statement: "Public health officials should get the names of the sexual partners of people who have tested positive for the AIDS virus so they can be traced and notified." Another 15 percent agree somewhat.

Effectiveness of AIDS Programs. We also asked respondents to rate the effectiveness of programs aimed at reducing the spread of AIDS through education and voluntary testing across a variety of different target groups. Although the majority of respondents perceive such programs to be either somewhat or very effective, the level of effectiveness is rated somewhat differently according to the target group. Programs aimed at women of childbearing age were thought to be somewhat to very effective by 96 percent of the respondents, whereas the figure for programs aimed at teenagers was 93 percent and for gay/bisexual men it was 90 percent. In comparison, programs aimed at prostitutes and hustlers were thought to be somewhat or very effective by 70 percent of the respondents, and programs aimed at IV drug users by 59 percent (Fig. 4).

Public Priorities for Allocating Public Funds Spent on AIDS. We asked respondents to assume that they had $100 of public funds to spend on the AIDS epidemic and that they could allocate those funds according to what they thought was most important and where they thought the funds would do the most good. Given three choices—research on causes and cures of AIDS, treatment of people who already have AIDS, and prevention programs aimed at educating people on how to avoid getting AIDS—respondents wanted to spend most of the public funds allocated to AIDS on research (45 percent) and prevention (29 percent), with 25 percent for treatment (Fig. 5).

It is obvious that public perception about appropriate spending priorities differs from actual present and likely future spending distributions, in which treatment absorbs most of the funds available.[66] This is supported, at least in part, by the apparent belief in the need for and effectiveness of AIDS education/prevention programs.

---

[66]Actual spending distributions only partly reflect policy choices. Spending on treatment, for example, is governed by private decisions and by blanket entitlements under Medicaid and the Veterans Administration and does not reflect a simple decision to allocate some portion of a pool of flexible resources to treatment.

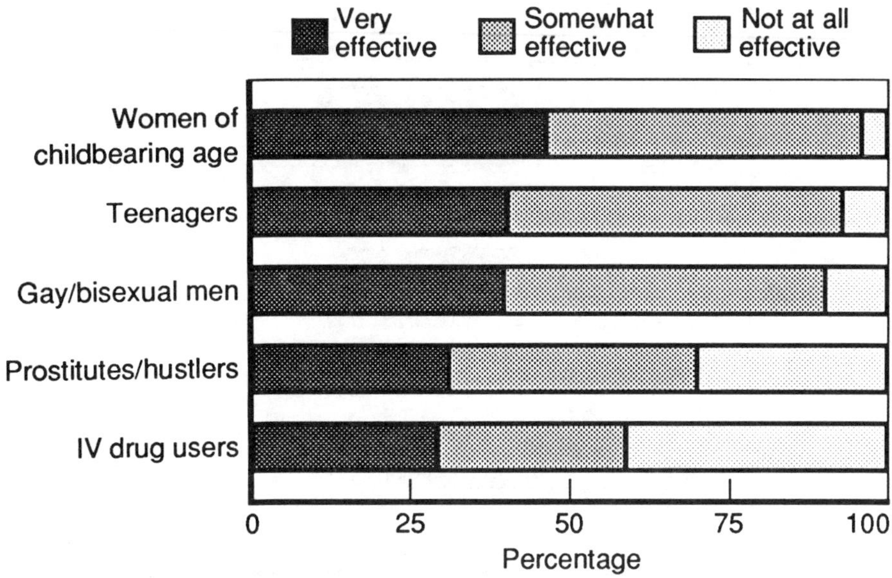

NOTE: Asked of all respondents (n = 1,305). Percentages exclude from 13 to 24 respondents who indicated that they did not know how they would rate the effectiveness of some of these programs and one who refused to answer the question.

Fig. 4—Percentage distribution of respondents' perceptions of the effectiveness of prevention programs for different target groups

HIV ANTIBODY TESTING

The Centers for Disease Control (CDC) funds 63 HIV prevention programs with testing centers through health departments in all 50 states, as well as in four cities, seven territories, the District of Columbia, and Puerto Rico. These programs have cumulatively performed approximately 2.5 million HIV antibody tests from 1985 to 1989 (CDC, 1990b). Of the roughly one million of these tests that are accompanied by information about the risk category in which the test-taker falls (e.g., gay/bisexual or intravenous drug user), nearly three-quarters (73 percent) are from heterosexual transmission categories.[67]

[67]The heterosexual transmission categories include the sexual partners of at-risk or HIV-infected individuals, heterosexuals with multiple sexual partners, and heterosexuals with other behavioral factors that led public health officials to classify these individuals as posing a heterosexual risk of HIV transmission (of all of those tested in these heterosexual transmission categories, 1.7 percent were found to be seropositive).

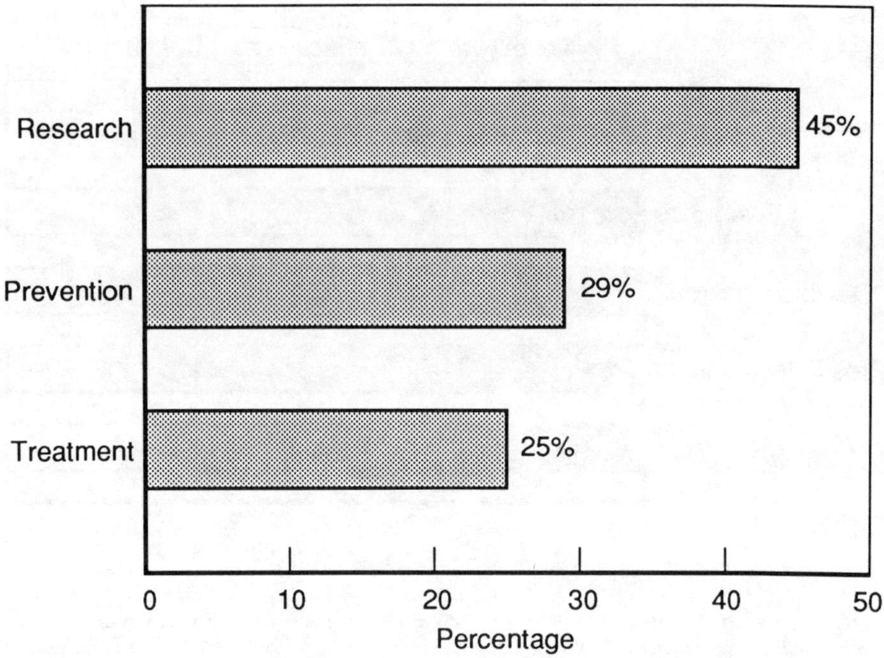

NOTE: Asked of all respondents (n = 1,305). Percentages exclude six respondents who did not know how they would allocate funds for AIDS.

Fig. 5—How respondents would allocate funds to AIDS

Even if the reported percentage of tests from individuals at heterosexual risk of HIV transmission is heavily discounted to allow for biased reporting, repeat tests, and differential use of confidential compared with anonymous testing,[68] these results suggest that there are many people who see themselves as being at risk of HIV transmission solely from heterosexual activity and who are actively

Heterosexual transmission also includes a group described as "other heterosexuals" with no history of risk behavior or no partner(s) identified as being at risk or actually HIV infected (with 2.3 percent being HIV seropositive). This category specifically excludes heterosexual intravenous drug users.

[68]For a discussion of how reporting and testing problems complicate attempts to estimate the number of people who have been tested, see Wenstrom and Zuidema (1989); Rhame and Maki (1989); Thompson (1989); Ohi et al. (1988); Fehrs et al. (1988); and Gostin et al. (1987).

seeking testing for reassurance or confirmation of their suspicions. Indeed, there has been a gradual shift in testing patterns over time, such that proportionately more lower-risk heterosexuals are now seeking HIV antibody testing (Danila et al., 1990; Beck et al., 1987).

It is inherently difficult to estimate population HIV seroprevalence rates based on the cumulation of data from different types of testing centers (e.g., alternative testing sites compared with sexually transmitted disease clinics) with different confidentiality requirements (e.g., anonymous compared with confidential testing). It is not clear what types of people use different kinds of testing facilities and how this might affect the observed prevalence of HIV infection in different geographic areas. Further, there may be important limitations in estimating HIV seroprevalence when an unknown number of people return for more than one test over time.

Although direct measures are, of course, not possible through a telephone survey, self-reports of HIV antibody testing from a systematically drawn probability sample of Los Angeles County residents[69] may be useful in illuminating how many and what kinds of people have been tested and what proportion acknowledge being HIV positive. We also asked respondents to estimate the likelihood that they would take the test in six months (if they had tested negative or had not already been tested) and to judge what the likely result would be if they were to take the test now.

Twenty-three percent of the respondents indicated that they had taken an HIV antibody test,[70] including those who had done so when donating blood.[71] This is somewhat higher than but still consistent with the proportion of adults estimated to have been tested for HIV antibodies in the United States (Hardy, 1990a, p. 9).[72] However, it is about four times as high as the 6 percent estimate obtained in a similar study that was conducted statewide by the California State

---

[69]We asked all respondents the HIV antibody testing series except for a small proportion who reported no sexual partners in the past ten years.

[70]The HIV antibody test was referred to as an AIDS test in the actual survey item. This wording is comparable to that used in the National Health Interview Survey and other surveys used among the general public.

[71]To discourage use of blood donations as an alternative way of getting tested, the American Red Cross has a policy of not providing results of HIV antibody screening to blood donors until three months after the donation has been made (if, that is, the results are positive; negative results are not reported to the donor). However, many respondents may reasonably assume that they are negative on the basis of never having been contacted after a routine blood donation.

[72]The National Health Interview Survey (NHIS), conducted from October to December 1989, found that 21 percent of the adults surveyed (weighted to represent the total U.S. civilian noninstitutionalized adult population) had been tested for HIV antibodies (including blood donors).

Department of Health Services Office of AIDS (Communication Technologies, 1988).[73]

To gauge the proportion who have actively sought testing (e.g., those using publicly funded county facilities or alternative testing sites compared with those using other locations) and those who have passively confirmed their HIV serological status through blood donations, we asked respondents about their blood donation history. Even though 46 percent reported that they had donated blood at least once in their lives, only 22 percent of the total sample[74] had done so in the last five years. It is therefore not surprising that only 18 percent of those who report having been tested cited the place where they donated blood as their testing location. The most common site for testing was the county testing sites, followed by private physicians' offices and research centers and hospitals (Fig. 6). More than eight out of ten respondents had only recently been tested (1988–1989), with what appears to be a near doubling of the number seeking testing every year that the test has been available (Table 23). The majority (63 percent) have taken the HIV antibody test only once, but duplicate tests have been taken by about one in every five test-takers (19 percent) and another 18 percent have taken three or more tests. With nearly 40 percent taking the HIV antibody test more than once, we explored whether this distribution was accounted for by very low-risk heterosexuals (parallel to the "worried well") or by people engaging in a variety of high-risk practices that justify a certain level of concern. We examined this question by conducting a multiple logistic regression evaluating demographic (including relationship type) and risk behavior predictors of getting tested more than once among those tested.

The only predictors significantly associated with getting tested for HIV antibodies more than once (Table A.12) were:

- Being male; and
- Being 35 to 44 years old.

---

[73]That study employed RDD sampling proportional to the number of households in each geographic area, including an augmented RDD sample within communities with denser minority representation for an oversample of black and Hispanic households. The study's purpose was to provide statewide estimates of HIV test-taking, beyond the epidemic's current focal points in San Francisco and Los Angeles. One would expect that the overall percentage of adults who have been tested statewide would be substantially lower than that found for Los Angeles County alone.

[74]Forty-eight percent of those who have ever donated blood (last donations ranging from 1935 to 1989) had donated from 1985 to 1989 when HIV antibody screening of the blood supply was being performed. This amounts to 22 percent of all respondents having donated blood at least once in the last five years.

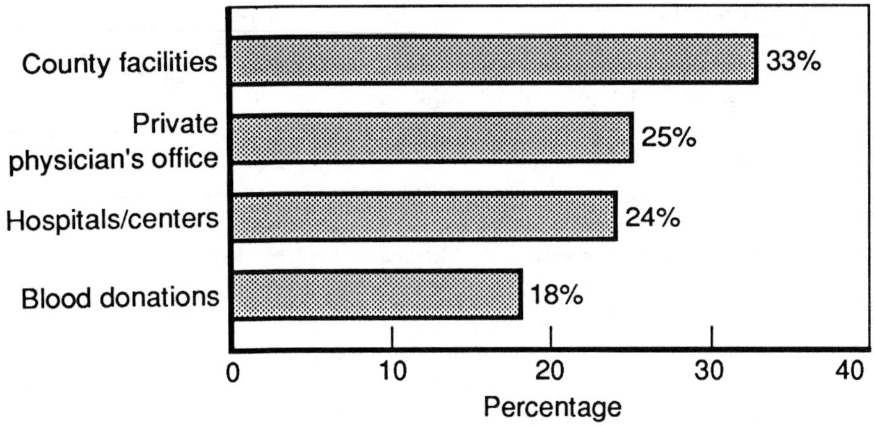

NOTE: Percentages based on the respondents who have ever been tested for HIV antibodies (n = 301), including those tested through blood donations.

Fig. 6—Where respondents get tested for HIV in Los Angeles County

Table 23

YEAR IN WHICH RESPONDENTS TOOK THE HIV ANTIBODY TEST

Year of Most Recent Test Taken	No. of Respondents	Percentage of Those Tested
1984	5	1
1985	6	2
1986	10	3
1987	41	13
1988	89	28
1989	147	53

These "risk factors" for undergoing multiple testing correspond to the age group and gender in which the greatest incidence of AIDS cases occurs. If these are the "worried well," then they are the "worried well" with the highest demographic risk profile. Surprisingly, however, being tested more frequently was not associated with engaging in high-risk behavior or with being in an open or nonexclusive relationship.

HIV Test Results

Of those respondents who had been tested for HIV antibodies, 0.3 percent (weighted to the county population) reported that their test results were positive. Another 0.2 percent never went back for their results. If all respondents who were not tested or did not get their results were HIV negative, this would suggest a low-end estimate of 0.1 percent HIV seropositive for the county as a whole (or roughly 8,000 HIV infected persons).[75] Since the cumulative number of reported AIDS cases in the county is substantially greater than that, this minimum is unrealistically low.

We asked respondents who had not been tested and those whose test results had shown them to be HIV negative what would be the likely result of an HIV antibody test taken at the time of the interview. Although 73 percent indicated that the result would certainly be negative, some 27 percent were less sure of that. If all those who thought that they would test positive were in fact positive, that would add another 0.7 percent of county residents to the pool of HIV infecteds.

Characteristics of Those Who Have Been Tested for HIV

We do not regard telephone survey data of the type collected in this study as providing a sound basis for estimating HIV seroprevalence. They are well suited, however, to answering an important question that bears on how seroprevalence data from voluntary testing can best be interpreted—namely, in what ways do those who seek testing differ from those who do not? We examined this question by looking at, for example, the demographic predictors of getting tested and not getting tested.

It is of considerable interest to examine the characteristics of those who have been tested and those who have not. To do this, we

---

[75]If the HIV positive self-reports are treated as valid and unbiased, they can be used to generate several population-based estimates of HIV seroprevalence. Each estimate, however, requires a different set of assumptions, any or all of which are questionable. The most conservative estimate of the HIV seroprevalence in the county would assume that all respondents who had not been tested were, in fact, HIV negative and that all of those who never obtained their results were also HIV negative. Although we do not believe these assumptions to be the most plausible that could be made, they do provide a low-end estimate of 0.1 percent HIV seropositivity (or roughly 8,000 HIV-infecteds in Los Angeles County if applied to the 1989 population). Estimates arrived at by other methods suggest that the actual number infected is much greater than that (from 55,000 to 112,000 HIV-infecteds according to the Los Angeles County Department of Health Services, AIDS Epidemiology Program), underscoring the problem of bias in survey-based approaches to estimating seroprevalence.

employed multiple logistic regression, including a series of possible demographic and AIDS-related predictors such as age, education, relationship status, and knowing someone with AIDS.

We found four variables significantly associated with getting tested for HIV antibodies (see Table A.13):

- Being under 55 years of age;
- Not having graduated from high school;
- Being married (to someone of the opposite sex); and
- Knowing one or more people who have AIDS.

The three demographic predictors suggest who may be most worried about being infected. Those under 55 years of age are more likely to have been sexually active outside their primary relationship since the start of the AIDS epidemic; those who are married may be especially concerned about transmission to (or from) their spouse; and those who have not graduated from high school may have a more diffuse concern about risks from casual contact. When we directly included knowledge measures in the model, however, they had no significant predictive value for who had been tested.

Knowing someone who has AIDS may increase the likelihood that an individual gets tested in several ways. First, those who have had sexual relations (or have shared needles) with that person, or who fear transmission through more casual modes of contact, may seek testing specifically as a result of that contact. With misperception of the risks of casual contact with someone with AIDS being relatively common, a portion of the respondents who "know" someone with AIDS may simply be dispelling their worst fears. Second, knowing someone with AIDS may increase the salience of the disease by providing a first-hand observation of its course and effects on one's contemporaries or acquaintances.

As the epidemic continues to grow, increasing numbers of people will know someone who is infected with HIV or has AIDS. Insofar as knowing someone with AIDS continues to motivate others to be tested, further increases in the demand for testing may occur.

Our results regarding the determinants of getting tested suggest that those who have sought HIV testing come from virtually all segments of the county's population, but they differ from the average county resident in important ways. They are less likely to be older, less likely to be high school graduates, and more likely to be married and to know someone with AIDS. But use of testing services is by no means limited to the "worried well."

Unfortunately, we cannot use these cross-sectional data to examine testing patterns over time or to determine to what extent testing results (positive or negative) influence subsequent behavior.[76]

Likelihood of Taking the Test in the Future

We asked all respondents who had not been tested or who tested HIV negative how likely it was that they would take the HIV antibody test in the next six months. Forty percent said that it was somewhat to extremely likely that they would take it (Table 24). This provides further evidence that the demand for testing is likely to continue at a high level.

Table 24

RESPONDENTS' LIKELIHOOD OF TAKING THE HIV ANTIBODY TEST IN THE FUTURE

Likelihood of Taking Test in Next Six Months[a]	No. of Respondents	Percentage of Those Who Tested Negative or Had Never Been Tested
Extremely likely	82	7
Very likely	111	11
Moderately likely	97	9
Somewhat likely	168	13
Not at all likely	712	60

[a]Asked of 1,170 respondents who had not been tested or who tested negative. (Eleven respondents said they did not know how likely it was that they would get tested.)

[76]Other studies have addressed the effects of known test results on gay and bisexual men. See, for example, Coates et al. (1988) and McCusker et al. (1988).

IV. CONCLUSIONS AND POLICY IMPLICATIONS

In this final section we put our findings in context and discuss their implications for policy and for future research.

This study yields three main findings:

- The overwhelming majority of adult county residents do not behave in ways that place them at risk of becoming infected with HIV.
- Virtually everyone over the age of 18 in Los Angeles County now knows how HIV is transmitted.
- Many people still overestimate the risks of transmission through casual contact.

These findings have several implications for public policy:

- Efforts to change risky behavior should be directed as much as possible at the specific groups that are most likely to engage in such behavior.
- The most useful new information is likely to be gained by directing future research efforts at understanding the behavior of high-risk groups and how to change it rather than by conducting further studies of the risk behavior of the general population.
- AIDS education of the broad population should place increased emphasis on (1) correcting persistent misperceptions about the risk of casual transmission and (2) maintaining public awareness of the major ways HIV is transmitted and how people can avoid becoming infected.
- Most education programs should target specific groups: children and teenagers, for whom the information will often be new; those who are at elevated risk without their necessarily being aware of it (e.g., those with partners who are at high risk); and, of course, people who engage in high-risk behaviors without fully understanding the risks involved.

We believe that this survey closely represented residents in Los Angeles County and that most respondents reported candidly on the personal aspects of their lives addressed by the interview. But AIDS in Los Angeles County has not spread by the typical behavior of most people, as the results of this survey show. At any given time, the vast majority of adult county residents do not engage in behavior that would place them at high risk of HIV infection. Most are either monogamously involved in heterosexual relationships with a spouse or other partner who is unlikely to be infected by other partners, or else are sexually inactive. Although nearly all are concerned about AIDS as a public health issue, few seem to view it as a personal health threat, given their current behavior. In most cases, there is no particular reason why they should. Unless our survey data are at striking variance with actual behavior in the community (which we consider unlikely), they provide no evidence of an effective behavioral pathway by which HIV could quickly spread into that community on a large scale.

Instead, AIDS has spread within small subpopulations of the county and members of these subpopulations are probably underrepresented in this and most other general population surveys. Seroprevalence data suggest that the incidence of new HIV infections still concentrates in these subpopulations, whose geographic location, demographic characteristics, and behavior place them in the immediate path of the virus—for example, minorities in inner-city neighborhoods with high rates of IV drug use. In Los Angeles County, which does not have a large IV drug-using population that behaves in ways favoring HIV transmission, those in the gay and bisexual community have borne the highest risk, and that is likely to continue for some time.

Given that the risk is still so concentrated, it makes sense to focus prevention resources where they are still most urgently needed, targeting the subpopulations that face the greatest risk. New entrants to these high-risk populations seem especially important (e.g., young people, both gay and straight, who are just becoming sexually active).

Locating and reaching people at high risk is not necessarily easy. Like Los Angeles County itself, the epidemic will probably continue to be diffuse and multicentered. It may be well to use sexually transmitted disease surveillance data to pinpoint the communities and subpopulations in which HIV is most likely to be spreading. Data from military applicants indicate that geographic patterns tend to be quite stable over time, which suggests that the county's own AIDS surveillance data may provide the best record not only of past patterns of concentration but likely future ones as well.

Designing effective programs for specific groups is not easy. Very little research has been done to answer the basic questions that need to be answered to design effectively targeted interventions. Priority for future research funding should, in our view, be placed on imaginative but systematic studies of these high-risk subpopulations. These research results could be used to develop such interventions and provide the basis for evaluating them.

One of the most striking features of our results concerns the high level of knowledge exhibited by most county residents regarding the major ways in which HIV is transmitted. This is good news, of course, and a success story for a major effort at public health education conducted at both the national and local levels. But it does raise questions about how much more education is needed and where it should be directed.

We believe that there is a compelling need for continuing efforts to inform (and remind) the public about how HIV is transmitted and how infection can be avoided. The goal is no longer to provide new information to the public as a whole but rather to maintain the salience of an important public health message whose implications for individual behavior are obvious but all too easily ignored.

We find overwhelming public support for AIDS education in the schools at all levels above elementary school, and a strong majority supports education at the elementary level as well. Most of the public believes in the effectiveness of education and prevention programs targeted at specific groups and is willing to have a significant portion of AIDS funding allocated to prevention.

Our results also document continuing confusion and misperception regarding the risk of casual transmission, e.g., by means of food handling, coughing, and sneezing. Further, they suggest that these perceptions can have socially undesirable consequences; those who consider casual transmission possible express much less willingness to work with someone who has AIDS or is infected with HIV. Stepping up the effort to educate the public to correct these misperceptions could pay social dividends in the form of reduced discrimination toward people with AIDS.

Finally, our results show that the county's alternative HIV antibody testing program has been used extensively by those seeking testing. Such people are not limited to those in high-risk groups but form a broad cross-section of the county population. Married people, people with less than high school educations, and people under the age of 55 have been especially likely to seek testing. Judging from stated intentions of those who have not yet been tested, this demand is likely to continue at a high level.

Appendix

REGRESSION RESULTS

Table A.1

PREDICTORS OF ENGAGING IN ANY UNPROTECTED ANAL INTERCOURSE: RESULTS OF LOGISTIC REGRESSION

Variables	Coefficient	S.E.
Intercept	-1.20	1.95
Age 25–34	0.52	0.67
Age 35–44	0.38	0.74
Age 45–54	-0.08	0.78
Age 55+	-1.28	1.22
Male	1.55***	0.47
Black	-1.47	0.83
Hispanic	-0.51	0.59
Asian	0.41	0.71
Other race	0.62	0.87
High school graduate	-0.57	0.64
Some college	-1.62*	0.69
Household income (x1000)	0.01	0.01
Not employed	-1.18	0.78
Married (opposite sex)	1.40	0.72
Primary exclusive relationship	1.62*	0.72
Self-identified gay/bisexual man	2.10	1.27
Know someone with AIDS	-0.09	0.47
Knowledge/casual modes	-0.02*	0.01
Knowledge/noncasual modes	-0.02	0.01

NOTE: Direction of scoring of the dependent variable was reversed so that the sign of the coefficient would indicate the direction of the relationship.

*Coefficient significantly different from 0 with $p < 0.05$.

**Coefficient significantly different from 0 with $p < 0.01$.

***Coefficient significantly different from 0 with $p < 0.001$.

Table A.2

PREDICTORS OF FREQUENCY OF UNPROTECTED VAGINAL INTERCOURSE: RESULTS OF ORDINARY LEAST SQUARES REGRESSION

Variables	Coefficient	S.E.	t
Intercept	–2.33	2.42	–0.97
Age 25–34	1.38	0.61	2.25*
Age 35–44	1.18	0.68	1.74
Age 45–54	0.16	0.72	0.22
Age 55+	–2.15	0.76	–2.83**
Male	1.44	0.41	3.50***
Black	–1.00	0.54	–1.84
Hispanic	–0.38	0.61	–0.62
Asian	–0.80	0.88	–0.91
Other race	–0.72	1.18	–0.61
High school graduate	–0.54	0.77	–0.70
Some college	–0.13	0.78	–0.17
Household income (x1000)	0.0070	0.0081	0.87
Not employed	–0.90	0.48	–1.88
Married (opposite sex)	3.72	0.50	7.49***
Primary exclusive relationship	3.82	0.56	6.83***
Self-identified gay/bisexual man	–4.87	2.22	–2.19*
Know someone with AIDS	0.61	0.42	1.45
Knowledge/casual modes	–0.0022	0.011	–0.20
Knowledge/noncasual modes	0.034	0.022	1.58

R-square = 0.155

*Coefficient significantly different from 0 with $p < 0.05$.
**Coefficient significantly different from 0 with $p < 0.01$.
***Coefficient significantly different from 0 with $p < 0.001$.

Table A.3

PREDICTORS OF FREQUENCY OF CONDOM USE: RESULTS OF ORDINARY LEAST SQUARES REGRESSION

Variables	Coefficient	S.E.	t
Intercept	3.04	0.70	4.36***
Age 25–34	0.33	0.18	1.80
Age 35–44	0.62	0.20	3.11**
Age 45–54	0.82	0.21	3.82***
Age 55+	0.88	0.23	3.85***
Male	–0.20	0.12	–1.61
Black	0.17	0.16	1.07
Hispanic	0.04	0.18	0.24
Asian	–0.05	0.26	–0.18
Other race	–0.18	0.36	–0.50
High school graduate	–0.13	0.23	–0.59
Some college	–0.32	0.23	–1.37
Household income (x1000)	0.0009	0.002	0.39
Not employed	–0.08	0.14	–0.55
Married (opposite sex)	1.15	0.15	7.65***
Primary exclusive relationship	0.48	0.17	2.87**
Self-identified gay/bisexual man	–0.51	0.66	–0.77
Know someone with AIDS	–0.11	0.13	–0.83
Knowledge/casual modes	0.0015	0.003	0.45
Knowledge/noncasual modes	0.0070	0.006	1.11
R-square = 0.145			

*Coefficient significantly different from 0 with $p < 0.05$.
**Coefficient significantly different from 0 with $p < 0.01$.
***Coefficient significantly different from 0 with $p < 0.001$.

Table A.4

PREDICTORS OF AIDS-RELATED KNOWLEDGE: RESULTS OF ORDINARY LEAST SQUARES REGRESSION

	Knowledge Regarding Noncasual Transmission			Knowledge Regarding Casual Transmission		
Variables	Coefficient	S.E.	t	Coefficient	S.E.	t
Intercept	93.18	1.51	61.71***	57.24	3.05	18.99***
Age 25–34	1.40	0.98	1.43	–0.18	1.88	–0.09
Age 35–44	2.86	1.07	2.66**	–0.54	2.07	–0.26
Age 45–54	1.76	1.15	1.53	–4.34	2.20	–1.97*
Age 55+	2.14	1.11	1.93	–2.74	2.16	–1.27
Male	–0.86	0.65	–1.34	2.30	1.25	1.04
Black	1.36	0.82	1.55	–15.34	1.48	–9.71***
Hispanic	–1.39	0.93	–1.49	–8.13	1.83	–4.44***
Asian	–2.82	1.38	–2.05*	–14.86	2.59	–5.73***
Other race	0.70	2.01	0.35	–13.03	3.72	–3.58***
High school graduate	3.10	1.10	2.83**	7.04	2.27	3.10***
Some college	2.82	1.11	2.55*	10.98	2.26	4.85***
Household income (x1000)	0.012	0.012	0.94	0.14	0.024	5.61***
Not employed	–0.79	0.73	–1.08	1.19	1.44	0.83
Married (opposite sex)	–0.31	0.74	–0.41	–3.94	1.46	–2.70**
Primary exclusive relation.	0.60	0.89	0.68	3.35	1.71	1.96
Self-identified gay/ bisexual man	–0.22	3.71	–0.06	11.35	6.77	1.68
Know someone with AIDS	–0.16	0.67	–0.24	4.08	1.29	3.17**
	R-square = 0.041			R-square = 0.252		

*Coefficient significantly different from 0 with p < 0.05.
**Coefficient significantly different from 0 with p > 0.01.
***Coefficient significantly different from 0 with p < 0.001.

Table A.5

PREDICTORS OF WHO USES TV OR RADIO AS A MAJOR SOURCE OF AIDS INFORMATION: RESULTS OF LOGISTIC REGRESSION

Variables	Coefficient	S.E.
Intercept	1.12**	0.34
Age 25–34	0.47*	0.21
Age 35–44	0.22	0.23
Age 45–54	0.68**	0.26
Age 55–64	−0.086	0.27
Age 65+	0.30	0.31
Male	0.23	0.15
Black	−0.03	0.18
Hispanic	0.12	0.21
Asian	−0.24	0.29
Other race	0.21	0.46
High school graduate	−0.15	0.27
Some college	−0.34	0.27
Household income (x1000)	−0.0056*	0.0027
Not employed	0.12	0.17
Married (opposite sex)	0.19	0.18
Primary exclusive relationship	−0.39*	0.20
Primary open relationship	−0.080	0.34

NOTE: n = 833. Direction of scoring of the dependent variable was reversed so that the sign of the coefficient would indicate the direction of the relationship.

*Coefficient significantly different from 0 with $p < 0.05$.

**Coefficient significantly different from 0 with $p < 0.01$.

***Coefficient significantly different from 0 with $p < 0.001$.

Table A.6

PREDICTORS OF WHO USES MAGAZINES/NEWSPAPERS AS A MAJOR SOURCE OF AIDS INFORMATION: RESULTS OF LOGISTIC REGRESSION

Variables	Coefficient	S.E.
Intercept	−0.82**	0.31
Age 25–34	0.26	0.20
Age 35–44	0.50*	0.22
Age 45–54	1.06***	0.24
Age 55–64	0.89***	0.27
Age 65+	1.65***	0.31
Male	0.12	0.14
Black	−0.75***	0.17
Hispanic	−0.30	0.19
Asian	0.34	0.32
Other race	−0.71	0.41
High school graduate	0.30	0.22
Some college or more	0.98***	0.23
Household income (x1000)	0.00082	0.0026
Not employed	−0.037	0.15
Married (opposite sex)	0.30	0.16
Primary exclusive relation.	0.37[a]	0.19
Primary open relationship	0.086	0.32

NOTE: n = 675. Direction of scoring of the dependent variable was reversed so that the sign of the coefficient would indicate the direction of the relationship.

[a]p = 0.053

*Coefficient significantly different from 0 with p < 0.05.

**Coefficient significantly different from 0 with p < 0.01.

***Coefficient significantly different from 0 with p < 0.001.

Table A.7

PREDICTORS OF WHO USES PAMPHLETS/BROCHURES AS A MAJOR SOURCE OF AIDS INFORMATION: RESULTS OF LOGISTIC REGRESSION

Variables	Coefficient	S.E.
Intercept	–1.34***	0.34
Age 25–34	–0.07	0.21
Age 35–44	–0.17	0.23
Age 45–54	–0.53*	0.26
Age 55–64+	–0.19	0.28
Age 65+	–1.05**	0.37
Male	–0.16	0.15
Black	0.75***	0.18
Hispanic	0.46*	0.21
Asian	–0.34	0.35
Other race	0.53	0.43
High school graduate	0.24	0.25
Some college	0.35	0.25
Household income (x1000)	5.63×10^{-6}	0.0028
Not employed	–0.16	0.17
Married (opposite sex)	0.12	0.18
Primary exclusive relationship	0.17	0.20
Primary open relationship	–0.30	0.36

NOTE: n = 298. Direction of scoring of the dependent variable was reversed so that the sign of the coefficient would indicate the direction of the relationship.

*Coefficient significantly different from 0 with $p < 0.05$.

**Coefficient significantly different from 0 with $p < 0.01$.

***Coefficient significantly different from 0 with $p < 0.001$.

Table A.8

PREDICTORS OF WHO USES SCHOOL AS A MAJOR SOURCE OF AIDS INFORMATION: RESULTS OF LOGISTIC REGRESSION

Variables	Coefficient	S.E.
Intercept	-2.16***	0.59
Age 25–34	-1.91***	0.29
Age 35–44	-1.39***	0.30
Age 45–54	-2.59***	0.49
Age 55–64	-3.85***	1.02
Age 65+	-2.59***	0.63
Male	-0.06	0.22
Black	-0.22	0.30
Hispanic	-0.015	0.30
Asian	0.47	0.40
Other race	0.38	0.54
High school graduate	0.96	0.53
Some college	1.11*	0.53
Household income (x1000)	0.0046	0.0039
Not employed	0.37	0.25
Married (opposite sex)	-0.35	0.31
Primary exclusive relationship	0.78**	0.27
Primary open relationship	0.83[a]	0.43

NOTE: n = 121. Direction of scoring of the dependent variable was reversed so that the sign of the coefficient would indicate the direction of the relationship.

[a] $p = 0.052$

*Coefficient significantly different from 0 with $p < 0.05$.

**Coefficient significantly different from 0 with $p < 0.01$.

***Coefficient significantly different from 0 with $p < 0.001$.

Table A.9

PREDICTORS OF WHO USES FRIENDS OR RELATIVES AS A MAJOR SOURCE OF AIDS INFORMATION: RESULTS OF LOGISTIC REGRESSION

Variables	Coefficient	S.E.
Intercept	–0.59	0.40
Age 25–34	–0.067	0.27
Age 35–44	–0.060	0.30
Age 45–54	0.15	0.31
Age 55–64	0.16	0.34
Age 65+	–0.073	0.38
Male	–0.024	0.18
Black	–0.28	0.23
Hispanic	–0.47	0.27
Asian	–0.79	0.49
Other race	0.57	0.47
High school graduate	–0.63*	0.28
Some college	–0.95***	0.28
Household income (x1000)	–0.0012	0.0035
Not employed	–0.25	0.21
Married (opposite sex)	–0.19	0.21
Primary exclusive relationship	–0.49	0.27
Primary open relationship	0.68[a]	0.36

NOTE: n = 833. Direction of scoring of the dependent variable was reversed so that the sign of the coefficient would indicate the direction of the relationship.

[a]p = 0.059

*Coefficient significantly different from 0 with p < 0.05.

**Coefficient significantly different from 0 with p < 0.01.

***Coefficient significantly different from 0 with p < 0.001.

Table A.10

PREDICTORS OF WHO USES MEDICAL SOURCES AS A MAJOR SOURCE OF AIDS INFORMATION: RESULTS OF LOGISTIC REGRESSION

Variables	Coefficient	S.E.
Intercept	-2.07***	0.41
Age 25–34	0.53[a]	0.28
Age 35–44	0.57[a]	0.30
Age 45–54	0.60[a]	0.32
Age 55–64	0.64[a]	0.34
Age 65+	0.37	0.38
Male	-0.26	0.17
Black	0.34	0.21
Hispanic	0.19	0.25
Asian	0.16	0.35
Other race	-0.061	0.56
High school graduate	-0.19	0.29
Some college	0.13	0.29
Household income (x1000)	0.0046	0.0032
Not employed	-0.064	0.19
Married (opposite sex)	-0.20	0.20
Primary exclusive relationship	-0.44	0.25
Primary open relationship	-0.41	0.42

NOTE: n = 197. Direction of scoring of the dependent variable was reversed so that the sign of the coefficient would indicate the direction of the relationship.

[a]These age groups were borderline in terms of being statistically significantly more likely to use medical sources as compared with 18- to 24-year-olds ($p = 0.59$ to $p = 0.062$).

*Coefficient significantly different from 0 with $p < 0.05$.

**Coefficient significantly different from 0 with $p < 0.01$.

***Coefficient significantly different from 0 with $p < 0.001$.

Table A.11

PREDICTORS OF WILLINGNESS TO WORK WITH SOMEONE WITH AIDS: RESULTS OF ORDINARY LEAST SQUARES REGRESSION

Variables	Coefficient	S.E.	t
Intercept	1.67	0.22	7.53***
Age 25–34	-0.14	0.12	-1.18
Age 35–44	-0.14	0.13	-1.15
Age 45–54	-0.43	0.14	-3.12**
Age 55+	-0.24	0.13	-1.81
Male	-0.071	0.08	-0.90
Black	0.072	0.10	0.70
Hispanic	0.12	0.12	0.99
Asian	-0.076	0.17	-0.46
Other race	0.42	0.23	1.78
High school graduate	0.030	0.15	0.21
Some college	0.069	0.15	0.48
Household income (x1000)	-0.0015	0.0015	-1.00
Not employed	0.17	0.091	1.81
Knowledge of risks of casual contact	0.031	0.0020	15.21***
R-square = 0.24			

NOTE: n = 978.
*Coefficient significantly different from 0 with p < 0.05.
**Coefficient significantly different from 0 with p < 0.01.
***Coefficient significantly different from 0 with p < 0.001.

Table A.12

PREDICTORS OF HAVING BEEN TESTED FOR HIV ANTIBODIES MORE THAN ONCE: RESULTS OF LOGISTIC REGRESSION

Variables	Coefficient	S.E.
Intercept	–0.92	0.98
Age 25–34	0.034	0.44
Age 35–44	0.93*	0.47
Age 45–54	–0.28	0.53
Age 55+	–0.68	0.75
Male	0.71*	0.32
Black	0.10	0.39
Hispanic	0.027	0.45
Asian	0.32	0.68
Other race	–0.99	0.80
High school graduate	0.51	0.52
Some college	0.60	0.56
Household income (x1000)	–0.0063	0.0059
Not employed	0.41	0.37
Married (opposite sex)	–0.35	0.41
In primary exclusive relationship	–0.35	0.44
In primary open relationship	–1.26	0.78
Self-identified gay/bisexual man	–1.67	1.28
Know someone with AIDS	0.45	0.32
Has engaged in any anal sex	–0.46	0.71
Frequency of unprotected vaginal sex	0.03	0.027

NOTE: Direction of scoring of the dependent variable was reversed so that the sign of the coefficient would indicate the direction of the relationship.

*Coefficient significantly different from 0 with $p < 0.05$.

**Coefficient significantly different from 0 with $p < 0.01$.

***Coefficient significantly different from 0 with $p < 0.001$.

Table A.13

PREDICTORS OF HAVING BEEN TESTED FOR HIV ANTIBODIES: RESULTS OF LOGISTIC REGRESSION

Variables	Coefficient	S.E.
Intercept	–0.96	0.50
Age 25–34	–0.11	0.23
Age 35–44	–0.05	0.25
Age 45–54	–0.24	0.28
Age 55+	–1.46***	0.35
Male	0.28	0.16
Black	–0.11	0.21
Hispanic	0.02	0.22
Asian	–0.17	0.36
Other race	0.61	0.42
High school graduate	–0.70**	0.27
Some college	–0.57*	0.27
Household income (x1000)	–0.0026	0.0031
Not employed	0.10	0.18
Married (opposite sex)	0.51*	0.21
In primary exclusive relationship	0.38	0.23
In primary open relationship	0.28	0.38
Self-identified gay/bisexual man	1.22	0.79
Know someone with AIDS	0.32*	0.16
Has engaged in any anal sex	–0.25	0.36

NOTE: Direction of scoring of the dependent variables was reversed so that the sign of the coefficient would indicate the direction of the relationship.

*Coefficient significantly different from 0 with $p < 0.05$.

**Coefficient significantly different from 0 with $p < 0.01$.

***Coefficient significantly different from 0 with $p < 0.001$.

REFERENCES

Beck, E. J., D. G. Cunningham, V. W. Moss, J.R.W. Harris, A. J. Pinching, and D. J. Jeffries, "HIV Testing: Changing Trends at a Clinic for Sexually Transmitted Diseases in London," *British Medical Journal*, Vol. 295, 1987, pp. 191–193.

Becker, M. H., and J. G. Joseph, "AIDS and Behavioral Change: A Review," *American Journal of Public Health*, Vol. 78, 1988, pp. 394–410.

Berry, S. H., *Los Angeles Today and Tomorrow: Results of the Los Angeles 2000 Survey*, RAND, R-3705-LA2000, October 1988.

Biggar, R. J., L. A. Brinton, and M. D. Rosenthal, "Trends in the Number of Sexual Partners among American Women," *Journal of Acquired Immune Deficiency Syndromes*, Vol. 2, No. 5, 1989, pp. 497–502.

Capell, F. J., and G. Schiller, "Efficiency of General Population Screening for Persons at Elevated Risk of HIV Infection: Evidence from a Statewide Telephone Survey of California Adults," in Floyd J. Fowler, Jr. (ed.), *Health Survey Research Methods, National Center for Health Services Research and Health Care Technology Assessment, DHHS Publication No. (PHS) 89-3447*, September 1989, pp. 167–172.

Capell, F. J., and G. Schiller, "Incidence of Heterosexual Pairings Associated with Risk of Secondary HIV Transmission: Population-Based Estimates," presented at the Sixth International Conference on AIDS, San Francisco, 1990.

Capell, F. J., D. J. Vugia, M. J. Wilson, and V. Mordaunt, "Epidemiology of AIDS and HIV Among California Women," presented at the Sixth International Conference on AIDS, San Francisco, 1990.

Catania, J. A., D. R. Gibson, D. D. Chitwood, and T. J. Coates, "Methodological Problems in AIDS Behavioral Research: Influences of Measurement Error and Participation Bias in Studies of Sexual Behavior," *Psychological Bulletin*, Vol. 108, 1990a, pp. 339–362.

Catania, J. A., D. R. Gibson, B. Marin, T. J. Coates, and R. M. Greenblatt, "Response Bias in Assessing Sexual Behaviors Relevant to HIV Transmission," *Evaluation and Program Planning*, Vol. 13, 1990b, pp. 19–29.

Centers for Disease Control, "Estimates of HIV Prevalence and Projected AIDS Cases: Summary of a Workshop, October 31–November 1, 1989," *Morbidity and Mortality Weekly Report*, Vol. 39, 1990a, pp. 110–112, 117–119.

Centers for Disease Control, "Publicly Funding HIV Counseling and Testing—United States, 1985–1989," *Morbidity and Mortality Weekly Report*, Vol. 39, No. 9, 1990b, pp. 137–140.

Centers for Disease Control, "Pilot Study of a Househould Survey to Determine HIV Seroprevalence," *Morbidity and Mortality Weekly Report*, Vol. 40, No. 1, 1991, pp. 1–5.

Coates, T. J., R. D. Stall, S. M. Kegeles, B. Lo, S. F. Morin, and L. McKusick, "AIDS Antibody Testing: Will It Stop the Epidemic? Will It Help People Infected with HIV?" *American Psychologist*, Vol. 43, 1988, pp. 859–864.

Communication Technologies, Inc., *A Report on Planning for the AIDS Epidemic in California: A Population-Based Assessment of Knowledge, Attitudes, and Behavior*, Communication Technologies, Inc., San Francisco, 1988.

Danila, R. N., J. M. Shultz, M. T. Osterholm, K. Henry, M. L. Simpson, and K. L. MacDonald, "HIV-1 Counseling and Testing Sites, Minnesota: Analysis of Trends in Client Characteristics," *American Journal of Public Health*, Vol. 80, No. 4, 1990, pp. 419–422.

DeBuono, B. A., S. H. Zinner, M. Daamen, and W. M. McCormack, "Sexual Behavior of College Women in 1975, 1986, and 1989," *New England Journal of Medicine*, Vol. 322, No. 12, 1990, pp. 821–824.

Department of Commerce, *Statistical Abstract of the United States*, Bureau of the Census, Washington, D.C., 109th ed., 1989.

Edgar, T., S. L. Hammond, and V. S. Freimuth, "The Role of the Mass Media and Interpersonal Communication in Promoting AIDS-Related Behavioral Change," *AIDS and Public Policy Journal*, Vol. 4, No. 1, 1989, pp. 3–10.

Fehrs, L. J., L. R. Foster, V. Fox, D. Fleming, R. O. McAlister, S. Modesitt, and R. Conrad, "Trial of Anonymous vs. Confidential HIV Tests," *Lancet*, Vol. 2, No. 8607, 1988, pp. 379–382.

Freeman, H. E., K. Montgomery, C. E. Lewis, and C. R. Corey, "Use of Telephone Surveys in AIDS-Related Community Research," in F. J. Fowler, Jr. (ed.), *Health Survey Research Methods*, National Center for Health Services Research and Health Care Technology Assessment, DHHS Publication No. (PHS) 89-3447, September 1989, pp. 173–179.

Gostin, L. O., W. J. Curran, and M. E. Clark, "The Case against Compulsory Casefinding in Controlling AIDS—Testing, Screening and Reporting," *American Journal of Law and Medicine*, Vol. 12, No. 1, 1987, pp. 7–53.

Green, R., and J. Wiener, *Methodology in Sex Research*, Proceedings of an NIMH Conference Held in Chevy Chase, MD (DHHS Publication No. ADM 80-766), U.S. Government Printing Office, Washington, D.C., 1980.

Hardy, A., "AIDS Knowledge and Attitudes for October–December 1989," *Advance Data*, No. 186 (Advance Data from Vital and Health Statistics, No. 179), National Center for Health Statistics, Hyattsville, Maryland, June 1990a.

Hardy, A., "National Health Interview Survey Data on Adult Knowledge of AIDS in the United States," *Public Health Reports*, Vol. 105, No. 6, 1990b, pp. 629–634.

Hingson, R. W., L. Strunin, B. M. Berlin, and T. Heeren, "Beliefs About AIDS, Use of Alcohol and Drugs, and Unprotected Sex in Massachusetts Adolescents," *American Journal of Public Health*, Vol. 80, No. 3, 1990, pp. 295–299.

Joseph, J. G., S. B. Montgomery, C.-A. Emmons, R. C. Kessler, D. G. Ostrow, C. B. Wortman, K. O'Brien, M. Eller, and S. Eshleman, "Magnitudes and Determinants of Behavioral Risk Reduction: Longitudinal Analyses of a Cohort at Risk for AIDS," *Psychology and Health*, Vol. 1, 1987, pp. 73–96.

Kanouse, D. E., S. H. Berry, E. M. Gorman, E. M. Yano, and S. Carson, *Response to the AIDS Epidemic: A Survey of Homosexual and Bisexual Men in Los Angeles County*, RAND, R-4031-LACH, 1991.

Kappel, S., R. L. Vogt, M. Brozicevic, and D. Kutzko, "AIDS Attitudes and Knowledge Among Adults in Vermont," *Public Health Reports*, Vol. 104, No. 4, 1989, pp. 388–391.

Kelly, J. A., J. S. St. Lawrence, H. V. Hood, and T. L. Brasfield, "Behavioral Intervention to Reduce AIDS Risk Activities," *Journal of Consulting and Clinical Psychology*, Vol. 57, No. 1, 1989, pp. 60–67.

Kinsey, A. C., W. B. Pomeroy, and C. E. Martin, *Sexual Behavior in the Human Male*, W. B. Saunders, Philadelphia, 1948.

Landefeld, C. S., M. M. Chren, J. Shega, T. Speroff, and E. McGuire, "Students' Sexual Behavior, Knowledge, and Attitudes Relating to the Acquired Immunodeficiency Syndrome," *Journal of General Internal Medicine*, Vol. 3, 1988, pp. 161–165.

Leigh, B. C., "The Relationship of Substance Use During Sex to High-Risk Sexual Behavior," *The Journal of Sex Research*, Vol. 27, 1990, pp. 199–213.

Longshore, D., and M. D. Anglin, *HIV Seroprevalence and AIDS Risk Among Drug Users in Los Angeles County*, paper prepared for the AIDS Program Office, Los Angeles County, by the Drug Abuse Research Group, University of California, Los Angeles, December 1990.

Los Angeles County Department of Health Services, AIDS Epidemiology Program, Monthly Surveillance Report, December 31, 1990.

McCusker, J., A. M. Stoddard, K. H. Mayer, J. Zapka, C. Morrison, and S. P. Saltzman, "Effects of HIV Antibody Test Knowledge on Subsequent Sexual Behaviors in a Cohort of Homosexually Active Men," *American Journal of Public Health*, Vol. 78, 1988, pp. 462–467.

Miller, H. G., C. F. Turner, and L. E. Moses, "Methodological Issues in AIDS Surveys," chapter 6 in *AIDS: The Second Decade*, National Academy Press, Washington, D.C., 1990, pp. 359–471.

Minkoff, H., S. McKalla, I. Delke, J. Feldman, R. Stevens, and M. Salwen, "Cocaine Use and Sexually Transmitted Diseases Including HIV," presented at the Fifth International Conference on AIDS, Montreal, 1989.

National Institute on Drug Abuse (NIDA), *National Household Survey on Drug Abuse: Main Findings 1988*, DHHS Publication No. (ADM) 90-1682, Rockville, Maryland, 1990.

Ohi, G., H. Terao, T. Hasegawa, W. Hirano, I. Kai, Y. Kobayashi, Y. Inaba, Y. Muramatsu, T. Miyama, M. Ashizawa, M. Kamakurea, I. Vemura, and T. Niimi, "Notification of HIV Carriers: Possible Effect on Uptake of AIDS Testing," *Lancet*, Vol. 2, 1988, pp. 947–949.

Pappaioanou, M., T. J. Dondero, L. R. Peterson, I. M. Onerato, C. D. Sanchez, and J. W. Curran, "The Family of HIV Seroprevalence Surveys: Objectives, Methods, and Uses of Sentinel Surveillance for HIV in the United States," *Public Health Reports*, Vol. 105, No. 2, 1990, pp. 113–119.

Research Triangle Institute (RTI), *National Household Seroprevalence Survey Feasibility Study Final Report*, Research Triangle Institute, Report No. RTI/4190-01-01F, Research Triangle Park, North Carolina, April 30, 1990.

Rhame, F. S., and D. G. Maki, "The Case for Wider Use of Testing for HIV Infections," *New England Journal of Medicine*, Vol. 320, No. 19, 1989, pp. 1248–1254.

Siegel, K., L. J. Bauman, G. H. Krist, and S. Krown, "Patterns of Change in Sexual Behavior among Gay Men in New York City," *Archives of Sexual Behavior*, Vol. 17, 1988, pp. 481–497.

Siegel, K., F. P. Mesagno, J. Y. Chen, and G. Christ, "Factors Distinguishing Homosexual Males Practicing Risky and Safer Sex," *Social Science and Medicine,* Vol. 28, 1989, pp. 561–569.

Stall, R., M. Ekstrand, L. Pollack, and T. J. Coates, "Relapse from Safer Sex: The AIDS Behavioral Research Project," presented at the Sixth International Conference on AIDS, San Francisco, 1990.

Stall, R. D., L. McKusick, J. Wiley, T. J. Coates, and D. G. Ostrow, "Alcohol and Drug Use During Sexual Activity and Compliance with Safe Sex Guidelines for AIDS: The AIDS Behavioral Research Project," *Health Education Quarterly*, Vol. 13, 1986, pp. 359–371.

Stipp, H., and D. Kerr, "Determinants of Public Opinion about AIDS," *Public Opinion Quarterly*, Vol. 53, 1989, pp. 98–106.

Thompson, V. M., "AIDS Testing: An Economic Assessment of Evolving Public Policy," *Economic Inquiry*, Vol. 27, No. 2, 1989, pp. 259–270.

Turner, C. F., H. G. Miller, and L. F. Barker, "AIDS Research and the Behavioral and Social Sciences," in R. Kulstad (ed.), *AIDS 1988: AAAS Symposium Papers*, American Association for the Advancement of Science, Washington, D.C., 1989a.

Turner, C., H. Miller, and L. Moses, *AIDS, Sexual Behavior, and Intravenous Drug Use,* National Academy Press, Washington, D.C., 1989b.

Valdiserri, R. O., D. Lyter, L. C. Leviton, C. M. Callahan, L. A. Kingsley, and C. R. Renaldo, "Variables Influencing Condom Use in a Cohort of Gay and Bisexual Men," *American Journal of Public Health,* Vol. 78, 1988, pp. 801–805.

Watters, J. K., "Observations on the Importance of Social Context in HIV Transmission among Intravenous Drug Users," *Journal of Drug Issues*, Vol. 19, 1989, pp. 9–26.

Wenstrom, K. D., and L. J. Zuidema, "Determination of the Seroprevalence of HIV Infection in Gravidas by Non-Anonymous vs. Anonymous Testing," *Obstetrics and Gynecology*, Vol. 74, 1989, pp. 558–566.

Wyatt, G. E., "The Sexual Abuse of Afro-American and White American Women in Childhood," *Child Abuse and Neglect*, Vol. 9, 1985, pp. 507–519.